The Political Cost of AIDS in Africa

An Overview

Kondwani Chirambo

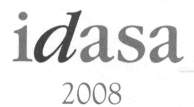

2008

Published by Idasa, 357 Visagie Street, Pretoria 0001

© Idasa 2008
ISBN 978-1-920118-66-2

First published 2008

Edited by Lois Henderson
Cover by Marco Franzoso
Layout by Bronwen Müller
Production by Idasa Publishing

Bound and printed by Logo Print, Cape Town

ACKNOWLEDGMENTS

The exploratory studies conceptualised, undertaken and led by the Governance and AIDS Programme (GAP) of Idasa over the past five years clearly revealed the relationship between AIDS and democratic governance on the one hand, and the capacity deficits of many of our institutions irrespective of the epidemic on the other.

These studies are the culmination of a project that began in 2003 amidst scepticism concerning the subject matter and its relevance to the overall national responses to HIV/AIDS. Yet in many instances, when audiences were faced with speculative theories, the fascination with the outcomes became self-evident. It has taken time to register new waves of acknowledgement about the importance of the work and its relationship to traditional areas such as politics, human development and health.

Over the years, the work has expanded to cover seven countries: Botswana, Namibia, Malawi, Senegal, South Africa, Tanzania and Zambia.

This abridged volume comprises the overview of the research; its aim is to make the extensive body of findings available to a broader cross-section of readers. This volume can be read alone – but for detail and analysis of the case studies refer to the expanded comprehensive volume.

GAP is developing strategic approaches for political leaders/policy-makers as a contribution to the effective management of the pandemic.

In all the countries, Idasa worked with state entities and civil society organisations. I take this opportunity to underline that the work could not have been possible without the involvement and dedication of our local partners; the Center for Social Research (CSR) at the University of Malawi; the Namibia Institute for Democracy (NID); the Economic and Social Research Foundation in Tanzania (ESRF); the Foundation for Democratic Processes (FODEP) in Zambia; and the Institute for Environmental Sciences at the University of Cheik Anta Diop, Dakar, Senegal. The researchers from these partner agencies, all of them senior academics and practitioners, have – apart from undertaking the country-based research – played pivotal roles in mobilising local political figures in the wide-ranging national forums that informed the pre- and post-research phases of the multi-country studies.

Without the involvement of officials from government, political parties, national assemblies, electoral commissions, People Living with HIV/AIDS, election NGOs, research institutions and above all the donor agencies that financed it, this would have been an exercise in futility.

It is hence with immense gratitude that we extend our thanks to the Swedish International Development Cooperation Agency (SIDA), which financed this most comprehensive of all our studies in this area. The multi-country research published in the companion volume, *The Political Cost of AIDS in Africa: Evidence from Six Countries*, was a follow-up to a pilot study conducted in Zambia in 2003, which was funded by the Ford Foundation and subsequent research in South Africa undertaken in 2004/5 supported by the Rockefeller Brothers Fund (RBF).

The support of these three donor agencies has placed GAP at the helm of a new body of knowledge that establishes the empirical link between HIV/AIDS and democratic governance, using the electoral process as an entry point. Based on its groundbreaking research, GAP has begun a process of developing strategic approaches for political leaders/policy-makers as a contribution to the effective management of the pandemic.

We may recall that the AIDS and Elections Project was an initiative that emerged out of consultations with political agencies at the highest level, among them: the Electoral Commissions Forum of SADC Countries (SADC-ECF), senior representatives from the United Nations Development Programme (UNDP) and the Joint United Nations Programme on HIV/AIDS (UNAIDS) country offices, the SADC Parliamentary Forum, the SADC Health Sector Coordinating Unit, civil society and donor agencies and the presidency of South Africa represented by Former Deputy President Jacob Zuma.

The second Governance and AIDS Forum was held on 22-24 May 2007 in Cape Town to discuss the findings of the multi-country study and was opened by the then acting Minister of Health, Mr Jeff Radebe (Minister of Transport). It brought together technical experts from the SADC region and francophone West Africa to examine the outcomes and suggest initiatives that might galvanise targeted policy responses. Electoral commission directors from the regions, AIDS experts, finance ministry officials, political party leaders and government department officials from South Africa participated in the deliberations that commanded worldwide media coverage. In short, the contributions to this project have been many and varied.

Finally, let me sincerely thank the staff of Idasa-GAP for their dedication to addressing the deficits in the research published in the expanded companion volume through additional work and interviews. In particular, Josina Machel, Christele Diwouta and Justin Steyn played important roles in delivering a product that was as close to our original vision as possible. Marietjie Myburg lubricated our public communication in several innovative ways. Jennifer Dreyer, and before her Vasanthie Knaicker, managed our administrative processes with great efficiency.

Dr Anne Chikwana, formerly Idasa's Coordinator of the Afrobarometer project, assisted partners with useful directions and insights on the use of public opinion data. Ann Strode of the University of KwaZulu-Natal and Dr Khabele Matlosa of the Electoral Institute of Southern Africa (EISA) continued to play important roles at various stages of the studies. Paul Graham, the Chief Executive of Idasa, was always available to us to be consulted and to provide moral support.

If we have failed to acknowledge others whose valuable input we benefited from, we do so with sincere apologies.

Kondwani Chirambo,
Manager Idasa-GAP

PREFACE

Elections are not enough to establish a democracy. The African Charter on Democracy, Elections and Governance establishes 11 principles of democratic governance, not only "the holding of regular, transparent, free and fair elections" but also those dealing with gender equity, corruption, representation, participation, political parties and transparent state processes.

Nevertheless, without elections and the possibility that these bring for the alternation or renewal of leadership, accountability to citizens by leaders, public choice, and a culture of citizen initiative and ownership of political systems, democracy cannot exist.

Despite encouraging signs of a shift in many countries on our continent to multiparty electoral systems, democracy itself is nowhere guaranteed; fledgling multiparty states have had to contend with endemic poverty, social and political upheaval, assaults on civil liberty and other challenges to the emergent new order.

Idasa's Governance and AIDS Programme (GAP) recognises that HIV/AIDS can destabilise the institutions of democratic governance, especially in countries where they are new and vulnerable.

Until we can end HIV/AIDS, we will have to establish AIDS-resilient societies.

Idasa established GAP to assist countries affected by the disease to explore its impact on governance and to investigate the best forms of parliamentary representation for managing the disease. It has undertaken public research and engaged in conversations with a range of stakeholders, taking its investigation to the very heart of the problem – the effect of the disease on electoral officials, institutions, voters and elected leaders, in fact on the electoral process itself.

This research has been conducted publicly through a combination of investigative work and engagement with those affected and infected by the disease. It has both immediate policy implications and more general policy lessons. It also considers the general political and social consequences of the disease – for determining budget priorities, allocating resources, shaping economies and communities, and determining the quality of public services, amongst many others. In particular, it looks carefully at the consequences for electoral systems and election management, and for the administrations, contestants and voters without whom our societies degrade their democratic legitimacy and efficacy.

We have to accept for the moment that we cannot cure the disease. And while, with considerable difficulty, we can encourage individuals to protect themselves against infection and prevent others from contracting it, we still have to adapt our societies to deal with the millions of people who are already HIV-positive – through medication, nutrition, daily care, and social and individual wellbeing – and with the consequences of unnatural death rates amongst adults of child-rearing and socially productive ages.

Until we can end HIV/AIDS, and even in the period from a cure to the last infection, we will have to establish AIDS-resilient societies. This book is about what may need to be done in one very important area.

This work would not have been possible without the support of the Swedish International Development Cooperation Agency (SIDA), which financed much of the research in this study. Thanks are also due to the Ford Foundation and the Rockefeller Brothers Fund for their role in financing this work.

Idasa has been privileged to work with five partners in this project: the Center for Social Research at the University of Malawi, the Namibia Institute for Democracy, the Economic and Social Research Foundation in Tanzania, the Foundation for Democratic Processes in Zambia and the Institute for Environmental Sciences at the University of Cheik Anta Diop, Dakar, Senegal. Our heartfelt thanks to them as well.

Paul Graham
Executive Director, Idasa

CHAPTER ONE: INTRODUCTION

1. INTRODUCTION

The Political Cost of AIDS in Africa is an expedition into the unexplored realms of a pandemic that today poses an unprecedented development challenge to a continent seeking revival amidst the rigours of globalisation.

It is a journey that takes us into the inner sanctums of politics and the uneasy environment generated by AIDS therein. It is, in essence, a discussion that unravels the challenges to political participation experienced by ordinary citizens living with HIV/AIDS.

It is a study that quantifies both the political and economic costs associated with the loss of elected representatives and voters to AIDS; one that ultimately illustrates the threat posed by the pandemic to the sustenance of democratic institutions.

This book is an abridged version of a far more detailed study that presents observations and recommendations for possible reasoned[1] interventions, in the short and long term. That companion volume is the fourth and most comprehensive book produced by Idasa as part of a five-year undertaking to establish the impact of HIV/AIDS on the electoral process within the broader context of democratic governance.

We launched this study with a pilot in Zambia (Chirambo: 2003), following it up with a comprehensive exploration of South Africa (Strand; Matlosa; Strode & Chirambo: 2005) and a preliminary release of our multicountry synthesis report (Chirambo: 2006).

The study's outcomes, we hope, will have broader policy relevance not only to strategies dealing with HIV/AIDS, but also to initiatives on electoral system design.

Followers of our work in the fields of HIV/AIDS and governance will recall that it was slightly over four years ago that senior political leaders, technocrats, academics and policy specialists from 12 countries in southern Africa and intergovernmental organisations converged upon Cape Town to discuss the governance ramifications of the pandemic.

In many ways, the two and a half day conference, organised by the Governance and AIDS Programme (GAP) of Idasa and the United Nations Development Programme (UNDP), was the first serious attempt to move what some might have considered a highly academic subject to the policy arena with a clear intent to demystify the link between two seemingly unrelated fields.

Idasa facilitated a process of dialogue on the implications of AIDS for democratic governance at the conference dubbed the Governance and AIDS Forum (GAF) involving senior representatives of regional bodies such as the Southern African Development Community (SADC) Health Sector Coordinating Unit (SADC-HSCU), the SADC Electoral Commissions Forums (SADC-ECF), the SADC Parliamentary Forum, the UNDP, UNAIDS; the presidency in South Africa, donor agencies and research institutions.[2] Country-specific stakeholder meetings were held in Namibia, Malawi, Tanzania, South Africa, Senegal and Zambia in 2005/6 that included senior state and non-state actors. These were reference group meetings which served to validate findings and further regional input, leading to the second GAF held in Cape Town on 22-24 May 2007. These participatory processes were meant to engender wider "ownership" of the problem and a shared policy approach based on the outcomes.

The first GAF conference was subsumed by speculative theory issuing from academics and defence analysts from the United States who postulated a complete collapse of state systems in Africa, particularly since many countries on the continent seemed to fit into the World Bank's definition of "fragile states."[3] With its catastrophic consequences characterised by gradual decimation of the relatively younger, economically productive and often more educated segment of the population, US scholars envisaged AIDS as almost certainly likely to further weaken the pillars of democracy: the economy, political institutions and political culture.[4] This analysis failed to critically consider the hubs of resilience within African societies such as extended family and kinship systems, all of which, although overwhelmed, continue to be one of the reasons why our societies at the very basic level of human organisation, have held together.[5]

The second GAF was challenged to seek solutions as a demonstration of the resolve of the African states in responding to the threats posed by AIDS to political institutions based on the findings of 2003, 2005 and 2006. Significantly, the second GAF was driven by African scholars who provided much richer understandings of their own contexts and were moved to challenge western experiences and definitions of democratic governance.

One of the most critical issues to arise from the 2003 GAF was the need to investigate the impact of HIV/AIDS on political stability, particularly relating to the electoral process a key indicator of democratic governance. Raised by the SADC-ECF, this issue was one that had occupied debates in academic circles and within Idasa for some time before that.

2. POLICY RELEVANCE

There are three main factors that have stimulated interest by political decision-makers and academics in this project:

- Firstly, both topics – HIV/AIDS and electoral reform – are matters of public policy concern. Their interrelationship may begin to catalyse a new form of discourse on electoral engineering and on strategies against HIV/AIDS, particularly in high-prevalence countries. Several of the southern African countries, including Botswana, Namibia, Lesotho, Malawi, Mauritius, South Africa, Zimbabwe and Zambia, have been entertaining the reform of their electoral systems, largely inherited from British colonialism (Matlosa; 2004; EISA 2004).
- From an academic point of view, the research is ground-breaking and has added new knowledge to the understanding of HIV/AIDS and its dynamics and has also, on the other hand, challenged conventional analysis and studies on political processes.
- Finally, experts on democratisation consider the electoral process as a means to

improve AIDS policy because leaders with the right credentials could assume power and effectively address the crisis. It has also been assumed that problems of weak mandates of the winners might arise if too few people turn up at the polls due to illness, care-giving and deaths. Mass manipulation of electoral outcomes through ghost voting could also manifest, thus generating tensions and conflict. Concerns around instability therefore remain central to this discussion.

It may be unwise to conclude from this preamble that the interest in the two topics comes from a discursive culture that continues to embrace a sense of openness on both matters. The reality cannot be further from the truth. On the one hand, electoral reform has been mired in inexplicable self-interest by succeeding generations of politicians in several countries, with a tendency toward lethargy at critical points of constitutional reform. Except for Lesotho, where armed conflict after the highly disputed election results of 1998/9 led to significant reform to the electoral model, the other countries have undergone long, drawn-out and inconclusive constitutional processes.

Ostensibly, the need to reform is an idea born of disgruntlement from opposition parties, trade unions and civil societies seeking greater accountability, gender and ethnic diversity, and transparency in government.

> Electoral processes can be galvanised by many factors, including corruption.

In South Africa, the Congress of South African Trade Unions (Cosatu), a strategic liberation partner of the African National Congress (ANC), has been at the forefront of agitating for a transformation of the country's Proportional Representation (PR) system to a Mixed Member Proportional (MMP) or Parallel system because of concerns around lack of accountability on several fronts including health.[6] Put more succinctly, electoral processes can be galvanised by many factors, including fraudulent electoral management systems, corruption, and cultural, economic and political exclusions influenced by electoral systems that serve parochial ethnic/elitist needs. Hence, the incentive to seek reform would have been animated by considerations that have a much longer history than HIV/AIDS.

We cannot, at this juncture, determine whether research initiated by Idasa will catapult HIV/AIDS to the top of the list of priorities that are likely to influence the political trajectory of these debates. We can say, however, that influential regional and national entities, including the SADC-PF's Committee reviewing the Norms and Standards of Election Practice have engaged with these matters in their deliberations with Idasa and appear to take cognisance of the gravity of the situation.

Through these technical committees, we may begin to see a change in the manner in which HIV/AIDS is discussed in political circles despite the now evident denialism that permeates the corridors of power across the continent regarding disclosures.

Historically, official acknowledgement of the disease as a potential political problem rarely manifested even as the AIDS epidemic peaked in the early to mid-1990s. But as the 20th century drew to a close, policy actors began marginally to show a sense of worry about deaths amongst political leaders.

It is worth noting for instance that seven years ago, the UNDP/SADC Human

Development Report (2000) warned of "…the slow collapse of the political, social and economic systems in the worst affected countries if measures are not taken to mitigate the impact of AIDS. For example, in some of the worst affected countries, repeated by-elections and delays in court cases attributed to AIDS-related illnesses and deaths is on the increase posing a challenge to the fragile emerging democracies in the (Sub-Saharan African) region" (SADC/UNDP/SAPES, 2000: pp. 150-151).[7]

Despite this, HIV/AIDS still did not form part of the debate on electoral reform. Policy experts argue that in order to gain the attention of the policy-makers, issues raised for the national agenda need to significantly qualify as public emergencies. Wayne Parsons (2003), in explaining the models in agenda-setting developed by Cobb and Elder, posits that an issue for public discussion is generated by both internal and external "triggers".

Natural catastrophes, unanticipated human events, unfair distribution of resources, among others could constitute an array of "triggering devices." AIDS, we assert, is a catastrophe of scale and has been declared an "emergency" by several African countries requiring a public policy intervention,[8] therefore any unknown impacts of empirical significance is likely to be of value to the improvement of national responses.

This recognition of AIDS as a security matter is timely.

At a global political level, no less an authority than the United Nations (UN) acknowledges that HIV/AIDS presents a *governance and security* challenge and is therefore likely to affect the manner in which member states manage their political, economic and social affairs at all levels. (Hunter 2003; UNDP 2002; UNDP-HDR 2002; WHO/UNAIDS Global Report on HIV/AIDS; 2006).[9]

Explaining the complexity of the epidemic in this regard, Peter Piot, Executive Director of UNAIDS, describes AIDS as "a massive attack on global human security" and attributes the failure of governments to recognise this to the timeframe of years and decades that the epidemic takes to manifest. This recognition of AIDS as a security matter is timely as the notion of security has been expanded by UNDP from implying the absence of conflict to meaning all fundamental conditions that are needed for people to live safe, secure, healthy and productive lives.[10]

Similarly, electoral reform is certainly a matter of public or common concern over which governments engage civil society, opposition parties and donor communities. It is also triggered in part by requirements for equal and equitable representation and access to power and resources.[11] The status of both topics under review in terms of their policy import therefore cannot be in doubt.

For its part, Idasa links its research on AIDS and governance to the disciplines of the intended target groups, by demonstrating how the pandemic affects the decision-makers themselves and their constituencies. This approach underlines Sandra Braman's (2003: p.48) assertion that in order for policy-makers to appreciate the value of social science research, those in the profession must learn to link their work to the disciplines in which the policy-makers are trained or located. Not surprisingly, the choice of elections, the means by which state power is organised, has resonated positively with elected representatives.

In our research, we have focused on five key areas: electoral systems, electoral management and administration, parliamentary configuration, political parties and voter participation. The institutions and actors involved in the electoral process all play a significant role in most instances in democratic accountability and the stability of government.

We do not for a moment equate elections with democracy. We do nonetheless underline the centrality of elections to modern democracies and particularly to emergent democracies in Africa. We critically analyse the place of the institution of elections within the concept of governance and its normative cousin, democratic governance. Our initial impression is that AIDS has the potential to unsettle a number of the strategic democratic institutions, thereby also affecting governance: the non-hierarchical manner in which nations are expected to manage their political, economic and social affairs based on a set of values, policies and institutional arrangements that include state and non-state actors.

3. HYPOTHESIS, METHODOLOGY AND IMPEDIMENTS

The electoral process as defined in this study is characterised by rules, institutions and a set of political actors. All the key elements under study have a bearing on democratic governance, as will be expounded in this chapter. Our aim therefore is to respond to the question: What is the impact of HIV/AIDS on the electoral process in Africa?

To explore the question, the project has investigated the following areas of the electoral process:

- Electoral systems: Increased deaths amongst elected representatives will be financially demanding on the state as by-elections mount in countries employing Single Member Plurality (SMP) systems and Mixed Member Proportional (MMP) systems.
- Parliamentary configuration: Power shifts arising from AIDS-induced by-elections are being analysed. Weaker parties are likely to lose policy influence as they fail to recapture seats that are declared vacant following deaths amongst their elected representatives.
- Electoral management and administration: Loss of core staff and part-time support personnel may affect efficiency; raise re-training costs and affect institutional memory. The management of the voters' roll will be problematic because of so many dead voters
- Political parties: The potential impact on political leadership and organising capacities of political parties is being studied: succession, financial implications and support bases may all be affected by attrition due to AIDS amongst cadres, leaders and stalwarts.
- Voter and civic participation: Focus Group Discussions (FGDs) investigate the impact of sickness, stigma and discrimination on voter participation from the perspective of PLWHAs. Will people infected and affected by HIV/AIDS withdraw from elections for lack of enthusiasm, or due to a sense of hopelessness? Conversely, will it galvanise PLWHAs and other civil society actors to demand treatment and care as a right?

3.1 ELECTORAL SYSTEMS: THE LINK TO DEMOCRATIC GOVERNANCE AND HUMAN DEVELOPMENT

Defined as the mechanisms that translate votes cast into seats and power in parliament and other decision-making mechanisms, electoral systems influence who is elected, how they are elected and therefore who decides on our governance priorities (including AIDS policy). Researchers in this area (Reynolds et al: 2005; Matlosa et al: 2007) indicate that the electoral systems can influence the quality of governance, the inclusivity of policy decisions and the nature of democratic accountability fostered by the party system.

More recently, the works of Gassner, Onhiveros and Verardi (2005) show strong correlations between the electoral systems and human development based on their effect on social security and welfare spending. The researchers employed simple econometric techniques and used several definitions of human development. The authors reveal that in majoritarian systems such as the First-Past-The-Post (FPTP) system (which is constituency-based) politicians will channel their resources to the districts where they are likely to obtain the most votes. The study further shows that under the majoritarian systems politicians will be more targeted since competition is concentrated in constituencies or geographically determined zones. Conversely, proportional systems, characterised by large voting districts, register higher levels of human development given the ambition by politicians to appease diverse groups nationwide (ibid).

> "We find that countries which have proportional systems enjoy higher levels of human development than those with majoritarian ones, thanks to more re-distributive fiscal policies. We also find that when the degree of proportionality, based on electoral size, increases, so does human development" (Gassner, Onhiveros and Verardi; 2005; p. 1 para 1).

Human development relates mainly to *widening people's choices regarding the acquisition of knowledge, accessing resources and living long healthy lives*.[12] Human development is closely linked to concepts of governance as articulated in a variety of authoritative works. Governance underlines the importance of transparency, accountability and the participation of all (marginalised) persons in decisions that affect their well-being (SADC/UNDP/SAPES: 2000: DPRU; 2001).

Electoral systems will be one of the institutions in the governance superstructure that link the governed and the governors in respect of how they select their development blueprints through an election.

In theory therefore, electoral models will contribute to enhancing the principles of participation and accountability so citizen choices on education, employment and health, among others, may be expressed through representation in decision-making processes. It may hence be inferred that electoral systems are integral to good or democratic governance frameworks[13] and are also relevant to human development.

This obviously implies that the choice of an electoral model has much wider developmental implications than may be normally envisaged. The next few paragraphs explain how each one of the electoral systems works and how they may influence governance.

The four main types of electoral system employed in southern Africa (and Senegal) that have been investigated in terms of their vulnerability to HIV/AIDS by Idasa are as follows:

Table 1.1: Electoral systems	
Countries	Electoral system
Zambia	FPTP
South Africa	PR
Namibia	PR
Malawi	FPTP
Tanzania	FPTP
Senegal	Parallel system
Lesotho	MMP
Idasa 2007	

SINGLE MEMBER PLURALITY (SMP)

Popularly referred to as First-Past-The-Post (FPTP), this system is considered the simplest. The country is divided into electoral zones and political parties field one candidate each to compete for the constituency seat. Independent candidates in most cases can compete as well. The candidate who receives the most votes is declared victor (even if one does not obtain more votes than all the others combined). One of the key elements of this system is the requirement for a by-election or supplementary election to fill vacancies in the event that the elected representative dies, resigns or crosses the floor. There are seven SADC countries that operate the FPTP electoral system: Botswana, Malawi, Mauritius, Swaziland, Tanzania, Zambia and Zimbabwe, most of which are former British colonies.

In the FPTP system, political parties tend to be personality-based, without clear policy and ideological direction and it's the strongest candidates (representing political parties or standing as independents), in the end, that claim a presence at constituency and national levels. The FPTP or SMP system is relatively stronger on accountability as leaders are directly elected by the voters and may lose power in succeeding polls if their performance is judged as poor. There is a range of criticisms directed at the SMP which include:

- Wasted votes, as losers' total votes will not translate into any form of representation;
- The translation of votes to seats tends to be disproportional;
- The system may disadvantage ethnic minorities as it's a game of numbers: small parties and women will also find it difficult to win in highly polarised and patriarchal environments;

- It often leads to a de-facto bi-party system;[14]
- On the basis of the work of Gassner, Onhiveros and Verardi (2005), we may add the relatively lower human development impacts observed under this system.

It can be argued therefore that the choice of electoral system allows for a particular class or section of society to access power and decide on AIDS priorities. Depending on the choice of system, decisions on AIDS could be representative of wider societal concerns or they could be decided on by a dominant ethnic group to the exclusion of minority considerations on the epidemic.

SINGLE MEMBER MAJORITY (SMM)

The Single Member Majority (SMM) system is similar to the SMP in that the country is divided into electoral constituencies. However, the fundamental characteristic is that candidates will be required to garner an absolute majority of votes (50 + 1 %) in the constituency to be declared winner. Sometimes, where candidates fail to achieve an absolute majority, a run-off is called. The SMM has been used for presidential elections in some countries in the Southern African Development Community (SADC) region, such as Angola.

PROPORTIONAL REPRESENTATION (PR)

Global trends suggest that Proportional Representation (PR) systems are gaining in popularity as they contribute to conflict resolution through their inclusive nature, and are therefore being touted as a means for democracy consolidation (Matlosa, et al: 2007). There are various types of PR systems practised worldwide; but the commonly used variant is the closed party list system. Under this system, the entire country is considered a single constituency. Political parties will contest this space and will be allocated seats according to the proportion of votes they obtain nationally. For example, a party that wins 40% of the total votes casts will theoretically secure 40% of the seats in Parliament.

> Global trends suggest PR systems are gaining in popularity.

The parties will use the closed lists submitted to the Electoral Management Body (EMB) to assign MPs to seats in hierarchical order. There is no requirement for a by-election when a vacancy occurs. Rather, parties will be allowed to fill the void with the next person on the party list. Angola, Mozambique, Namibia and South Africa are the countries in the SADC that apply the PR model.

Experts posit that PR models often encourage the formation of policy-based political parties. This is because, inevitably, the competing organisations need to appeal to the various interest and ethnic groups within the population to garner a decent percentage of the national vote that could translate into a proportional number of seats in parliament. Some of its strengths include:

- Encouraging gender diversity as women can be deliberately infused on to party lists for parliament;
- Promotes conflict resolution as minority parties will have an opportunity to gain a

foothold in Parliament, particularly when there is a low minimum threshold;
- Encourages the formation of parties or like-minded groups of candidates who will inevitably develop strategic visions to secure national appeal;
- Every vote counts; very few are wasted. With low thresholds, nearly every vote contributes to electing a candidate;
- Encourages nation-wide campaigns as opposed to parties restricting themselves to (ethnic or traditional) strongholds;
- Power-sharing between parties is encouraged;
- Tends toward longevity and stability of government as power configurations will not constantly change due to by-election losses, for instance;
- Higher levels of human development have been attributed to the PR system.

The PR system's weaknesses, in the eyes of most of its critics, are its tendency to:
- Build fragmented party systems and coalition governments which in turn lead to legislative "gridlocks" as representatives may not reach common ground on key issues;
- It may facilitate the presence in parliament of extremist parties;
- Voters cannot enforce accountability as the mandate to appoint MPs rests entirely with the elected party. There is no public input into who goes on to the closed party list;
- The PR system uses mathematical formulae which may be too complex for ordinary citizens to understand. The lack of appreciation of electoral systems is itself problematic in terms of the confidence it may generate in the long run (Reynolds et al: 2005; Matlosa et al: 2007).

3.1.1   MIXED SYSTEMS

Most countries will consider dealing with the short comings of either the FPTP or the PR systems by combining them into a mixed system. The Mixed Member Proportional (MMP) system and the Parallel system are both categorised as "mixed" but they do have their distinct differences, which are explained below.

MIXED MEMBER PROPORTIONAL (MMP)

It has to be underlined that while South Africa uses the PR system at national level, at local government level it employs the Mixed Member Proportional (MMP) system, which is a combination of the PR and FPTP systems. The system facilitates the election of one stream of Members of Parliament (MPs) or councillors through the FPTP system and the other through the PR system. In the MMP system any disproportionalities manifesting from the FPTP (or other) system is compensated for by the PR element. Only one SADC country, Lesotho, has adopted the MMP system at national level thus far (EISA: 2003).

THE PARALLEL SYSTEM

The Parallel system is also classified as a mixed system. However, the fundamental difference between it and the MMP system is that while in the latter the PR component compensates for disproportional outcomes from the FPTP (or other) system, in the Parallel model the two systems are independent of each other and are managed separately. In the SADC region Seychelles is the only country to apply the Parallel system.[15] In this study, Senegal is the only country to employ this model. Senegal changed its electoral system for the national parliament from list PR in 1978 to the current mixed, Parallel model which has been used since 1983 (Reynolds el at: 2005). There have been several modifications to the system.

3.2 THE POLITICAL SIGNIFICANCE OF AN ELECTORAL SYSTEM

Reynolds et al (IDEA: 2005) describes the choice of electoral system as one of the most important institutional decisions for a democracy because it has a significant impact on the political future of any country. It is an undertaking that should involve all stakeholders. And yet, its importance not withstanding, it is rare that electoral systems are in fact deliberately chosen. Influence from colonialism, neighbours or perhaps regional bodies might more often be the reason a particular model is chosen, he asserts. In instances where there is an opportunity for a measured approach to selecting an electoral system International IDEA proposes the following criteria:

- Providing representation: an electoral system must ensure that geographical representation, ideological divisions and party political situations are taken into account;
- Elections must be accessible and meaningful: People's votes must have a bearing on how the country is governed. Thus the choice of electoral system should influence the legitimacy of institutions;
- Facilitating stable and efficient government: The system must avoid discrimination against particular parties and interest groups; voters must perceive the system to be by and large fair;
- Providing incentives for reconciliation: Electoral systems must also serve as tools for conflict resolution within societies allowing for inclusivity of all ethnic and interest groups to the extent possible;
- Holding the government accountable: The system must facilitate accountability;
- Encouraging political parties: The system must be seen to encourage the growth of political parties, a key factor in the consolidation of democracy;
- Promoting legislative opposition and oversight: The electoral system should assist in ushering in a viable opposition which can exercise legislative oversight over government;
- Taking into account international standards: The system must embrace international covenants, instruments and treaties affecting political issues which form the principles of free, fair and periodic elections and which advance the principle of one person, one vote;
- Making the election process sustainable: The resources of a country must be taken into account. The availability of skills and financial resources are both paramount in operating an electoral system (Reynolds, et al, 2005).

This last point provides us an entry point into the discussion on AIDS as it relates to the sustainability of electoral models in the age of HIV/AIDS. Some of the countries discussed in the study seem to rely rather heavily on donor support in many sectors, including their electoral processes. Sustainability must almost certainly be one of the key considerations to be made in their electoral engineering undertakings.

3.2.1   PARLIAMENTS: POWER AND GENDER BALANCE

The operationalisation of electoral systems leads to representation and participation of various interests in decision-making mechanisms such as Parliament and local government. Depending on the system employed, there may be diversity or under-representation of certain segments of society. Often the aim of well-meaning nations is to ensure that the electoral system leads to fair outcomes, where the interests of the vast majority and minorities are expressed in the highest policy institutions.

> Organised women's groups have been used to assist female candidates in political parties to assume power.

We notice from a casual examination of the status of each Parliament in this study that countries using the PR have generally fared much better in gender balance compared to those employing plural/majority systems such as the SMM and FPTP. For the SADC countries, it was evident that only Angola, Mozambique, Namibia and South Africa attained the minimum threshold of 30% of women in decision-making mechanisms by 2005 a requirement of the SADC Declaration on Gender and Development of 1997.[16]

In the case of these four SADC states, women were deliberately infused into parliament, mainly by political parties weighting their lists of candidates toward the women in addition to having a gender quota within the party structures. The FPTP system will often struggle to meet these requirements as there can be no guarantee that a party with a relatively good gender balance will succeed in getting all or some of its female candidates into power through competitive elections. Patriarchal biases creep into both primary processes within party structures and amongst the electorate during campaigns. Maintaining the gender status quo once female candidates are lost to disease or other causes is highly unlikely in these circumstances.

Organised women's groups in some countries have been used to assist female candidates in political parties to assume power. In Zambia, in the 2001 general elections, the Zambia National Women's Lobby Group (ZNWLG) campaigned in favour of women candidates with some measure of success but not enough to infuse any form of gender equity (Chirambo et al, 2002). Out of the 198 women nominated by their parties to stand as candidates in the parliamentary elections only 19 won seats in the 158-seat parliament. (The total parliament size is 158 seats: 150 are elective with 8 being non-elective seats.) Compared to 1996 when only 59 women contested parliamentary positions, this was seen as an improvement in women's attempts to claim their place in decision-making processes.[17]

In Senegal in 1994, women drawn from politics, trade unions and activist groups banded together to form the Council of Senegalese Women (COSW). In the 1998 legislative elections the COSW launched strong female empowerment campaigns across all political parties and directed at parties, the media and the public. The resultant pressure pushed some political parties to institute 25% to 40% quota systems for women representatives. Although a bill was introduced by government in 2007 to provide for half of all candidates on the party lists presented by political parties to be women, the judiciary declared it unconstitutional. The exclusionary tendencies in the Senegalese system, it is argued in that country's chapter, are latent and inherited from French colonialism.

Tanzania's electoral model, while described as FPTP, has a legislated gender quota which is accessed through the PR model. Because of this, Tanzania has also been able to achieve the 30% threshold. There is, therefore, a need to stress the importance of the electoral system in configuring power in this regard.

Many experts will agree that representation in parliament can influence the way policy matters are prioritised. We noted earlier that vacancies in the FPTP system are filled through new competitive elections or by-elections, regardless of whether they occur as a result of an MP resigning, being dismissed or dying. In this study therefore, we are interested in establishing whether the frequency of by-elections, some of which may be caused by HIV/AIDS, necessarily leads to power shifts in parliament, with weaker parties failing to retain the seats they previously held. Do parties end up losing policy influence?

3.2.2   ELECTORAL MANAGEMENT AND ADMINISTRATION

LEGAL AND CONSTITUTIONAL FRAMEWORK

It is a well-documented fact that the overall integrity of any election hinges, to a large extent, on the legal framework and the uprightness of the institutions that conduct the polls. The legal framework consists of constitutional provisions, electoral acts and regulations or statutory instruments constituting such acts. Electoral procedures, the conduct of elections and the institutions that administer them are pre-determined within this framework.

Cognisant of this fact, the African Union, in its draft African Charter on Democracy, Elections and Governance, emphasises the need for the continent to develop independent electoral bodies. Chapter 7, Article 17 (1) of the Charter stipulates the requirement for member states to "establish and strengthen independent and impartial national electoral bodies responsible for the management of elections".

Prior to an election, there will often be two important processes that inform the management and administrative mechanisms in planning the poll. These are:
• The national census;
• Delimitation of boundaries.

The census: The national census is a survey of people resident in a country, which provides relevant data from national to community level. This information is essential for government planning, for business and for the community at large. The information establishes the demographic profile of the country, indicating how many people are citizens and how many of these are above or below voting age. Censuses have a long history dating back to ancient Egypt, China and Babylon when governments needed information so they could plan armies, as well as monumental projects such as the building of the pyramids or effect land re-distribution.[18]

Delimitation: Knowledge of population size and distribution enables the implementation of the delimitation process or demarcation of constituencies. A delimitation commission will be established to draw the constituencies' boundaries by applying a stipulated formula which defines the average size of the electorate to be assigned to each constituency. The demarcation of constituency boundaries is extremely sensitive and can be a source of post election conflict.

> **Electoral commissions are often accused of lacking independence.**

It is possible for governments in countries using the FPTP system for instance to re-engineer the boundaries, that is create more constituencies in areas in which the party in power enjoys majority support, therefore enabling it to get a larger proportion of the parliamentary seats. The SADC Parliamentary Forum (SADC-PF), which has a long history of election observation in Africa and has been used by both the executive arms of the SADC and the AU as a reference point in developing their charters, does take note of this and recommends that the impartiality of delimitation commissions in drawing up boundaries be re-affirmed in the constitutions of SADC countries. A number of key steps are suggested:

- The tenure of office of the commissioners should be guaranteed in the constitution;
- There should be no political interference in the demarcation of boundaries. The exercise should be left to the technical competence of the boundary delimitation commission;
- The commission should consult stakeholders in the process;
- Gerrymandering must be outlawed;
- Recommendations of the boundary delimitation commission should not be altered by any stakeholder.[19]

3.3 ELECTORAL COMMISSIONS

The information from the delimitation commission will in turn inform the management and administrative processes of the electoral commission. Electoral commissions lie at the heart of a stable democracy, lending credibility and integrity to the democratic process by ensuring that the rules are applied fairly; and that to the extent possible, the majority of citizens participate in freely making their choice of policy. In practice, electoral commissions are often accused of lacking independence, particularly since the government of the day or the president may have a hand in confirming nominations of commissioners or appointing them. Controversies surrounding electoral outcomes will not usually spare the electoral management body, hence the need to evolve a widely acceptable system of selection and appointment of chief electoral administrators and supervisors.

Recommendations from the SADC and the AU emphasise the need to avoid political interference from the executive in putting electoral commissions in place. Some of the recommendations by the SADC-PF include:

- The complete independence and impartiality of the electoral commission in dealing with all political parties should be re-affirmed in the constitution;
- Selection of commissioners should be done by a panel of judges set up by the Chief Justice or the equivalent "on the basis of the individual's calibre, stature, public respect, competence, impartiality and their knowledge of elections and political development processes";
- Selection of commissioners should be done in consultation with all political parties and stakeholders with final approval coming from parliament;
- The commission should have financial autonomy i.e. with its own budget directly voted for by parliament (and not allocated by the ministry of finance or any government department);
- The electoral law should empower the commission to recruit and dismiss its own staff based on professional considerations, rather than hire public service workers whose loyalty to the commission is not guaranteed;
- Electoral commissioners should have security of tenure entrenched in the constitutions of SADC states.

It is interesting to note that the recommendations imply an electoral process can be undermined by the manner in which a management mechanism is put in place or lack of consultation with other stakeholders or even by lack of financial autonomy, among other things. There is also evidently a move to depart from the use of temporary public workers as election officers because of potential accusations of partiality, depending on which department supplies the workers. If they are drawn from the office of the president, for instance, there are likely to be debates over the fairness of the outcomes.

The reality is that most Electoral Management Bodies (EMBs) do rely on the services of public service workers as support staff during elections anyway. Except for Namibia (among the countries we have studied), these countries from time to time enlist the services of public workers, particularly teachers and municipal workers. The aspirations of new democracies, we would imagine, would be to build the capacity of trained support staff over time to ensure that post-election conflict is minimised through diligent management. However, we do know from other authoritative studies that HIV/AIDS has been a major cause of deaths amongst public service workers, including teachers, and we ask therefore to what extent this form of attrition may undermine the management of elections.

CITIZEN AND VOTER REGISTRATION SYSTEMS

Lastly, the voters' roll is perhaps the most sensitive instrument in any election. It represents the aggregate number of registered voters and will ultimately serve as a key indicator of voter turnout. The representation of marginalised voices can also be extrapolated from voter databases, providing researchers, political parties, election monitors and others an opportunity to determine levels of political enthusiasm or validity of the data and ultimately the credibility of the electoral process.

In order to achieve this level of confidence, EMBs will need to have fairly sophisticated voter registration systems that will enable the removal of dead voters from the registers in good time before major elections. Knowing the size of the voter population before the poll is fundamental to allaying fears of fraud from opposition elements. To lubricate this process, states will need to institute citizen registration systems that are technologically compatible with the voters' rolls so that death certificates can be timeously processed and dead electors eliminated from the registers. The advent of AIDS may increase this work load for both home affairs ministries and EMBs. Worse still, countries without citizen registration systems or with outmoded systems are likely to struggle to cope with the number of deceased.

POLITICAL PARTIES

On the advent of independence or liberation most African states experienced the emergence of party systems dominated by the nationalist or liberation movements that existed at the time of achieving majority rule. With broad-based popular support for nationalist/liberation movements, opposition parties struggled to compete with the relatively more sophisticated rivals. In several of the countries in this study, including Malawi, Tanzania and Zambia, de facto one-party states were declared within ten years of independence from the British in the 1960s. This meant all official opposition was outlawed and the sum effect was that the party system was undermined even further (IDEA; 2000).

It was not until the early 1990s that a new wave of opposition emerged, usually breakaway groups from the founding party, to challenge those in power. Encouraged by relaxed registration rules, political parties began to make considerable contributions to democratic accountability, allowing for diverse interests to emerge. Studies by the United Nations Economic Commission for Africa (UNECA) indicate that in 2005, Chad had 73 political parties, South Africa 140, Mali 91, Ethiopia 79, Burkina Faso 47, Morocco, Nigeria and Botswana each 30, Egypt 17 and Ghana 10 (UNECA, 2005).

While there was a flood of parties, it has to be stated that experts noted the advantages of incumbency which placed ruling parties in a position to accentuate a de facto dominant-party system. This has been the case in Namibia, Botswana, Tanzania, Zimbabwe and South Africa. South Africa, with a PR electoral system at national level and state financing for political parties, has a relatively stable party environment as there seems to be an incentive to exist beyond elections. However, it is also characterised by a dominant party in the form of the ANC.

In most cases, political parties' performances will be determined in part by the nature of the electoral system. PR systems

Figure 1.1: Parties per Parliament

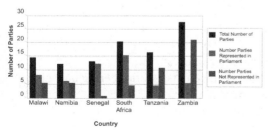

seem to reflect fairer outcomes while the FPTP system is often seen to present obstacles for the opposition, as discussed above. Party performances will also be determined by the amount of resources they have. Without a doubt, all parties would be assisted greatly if state funding was available without overly inhibiting pre-conditions. Malawi, Mozambique, Namibia, Seychelles, South Africa and Zimbabwe are some of the countries with state funding provisions for political parties.

There are however marked differences in the manner in which such funding is made available: in some countries the funding is restricted to election periods, while in others it is provided between and beyond the election period. The requirement in most cases for parties to qualify for funds is that they garner a prescribed number of seats in parliament. That being the case, it is hardly surprising that only one or two parties will in the end benefit from state resources. The level of funding available to a particular party will assist in levelling the playing field to some extent: they will be able to employ campaign staff, acquire transport to access the remotest parts of a country and deploy advertising in print and electronic media, as well as other communicative technologies (IDEA, 2000).

> Riddled with a range of institutional inadequacies, political parties may find epidemics such as HIV/AIDS weaken them further.

Because of the preconditions attached to accessing party funding, the reality is that launching a new party often means struggling against existing older parties in nearly all spheres. New parties will not have the organisational skills, finances or administrative systems to survive beyond an election or two. Often, they will also not have an ideology and will be guided simply by the desire to seek high office. While some of the current opposition parties were formally in power at independence, such as the United National Independence Party (UNIP) in Zambia and the Malawi Congress Party (MCP), most of them were formed in the early 1990s and will have narrow political bases (IDEA; 2000; UNECA, 2005). Most opposition political parties are headed by patrons who not only finance the institutions but also provide the leadership and they often have to close down after losing at the polls.

In Malawi for instance, of the nine parties that won parliamentary seats in the 2004 election, only three were more than ten years old. These were the Malawi Congress Party, the Alliance for Democracy and the United Democratic Front. The rest were created within three years of the 2004 election. In Zambia, nearly all the opposition parties that contested the second multi-party election in 1996 had collapsed by the time the country held its third election in 2001, except for UNIP which in fact boycotted the poll. Riddled with a range of institutional inadequacies, political parties may find epidemics such as HIV/AIDS weaken them further. There are three levels at which HIV/AIDS may impact on political party structures:

- Organisational: The loss of cadres and members affects electioneering capacity;
- Financial: Loss of members reduces subscriptions;
- Leadership: The loss of a patron may mean the end of a party or compromise electoral viability and financial status.

Without the support and participation of citizens, the legitimacy of our political systems is to be doubted. Our emphasis on citizen participation in governance processes in this regard was to determine to what extent, if at all, AIDS sickness and care-giving prevents people from adding their voices to the policy arena. Low participation can be problematic for democracies as issues of legitimacy creep in when too few people are involved in electing a government. Political scientists have warned about low participation in elections across the world for decades. Although turn-out as a percentage of registered voters in some cases may appear impressive, it can be disheartening when calculated as a percentage of eligible voters or the Voting Age Population (VAP).

Africa has not been spared this scrutiny and in several instances relatively low participation has been attributed to political disillusionment, poor incentives to vote, lack of service delivery by successive regimes, poverty, lack of transport, inaccessible terrain and the weather. Valid as these might seem, for a long time no consideration was given to AIDS as contributing factor.

If millions of people are ill, or are tending to sick relatives, surely they would be inclined to consider matters of personal survival ahead of attending a rally or standing in a long queue to elect a candidate for parliament unless of course there is a real belief that electing a particular candidate might dramatically usher in an era of better health care, non-discrimination in employment and accessing other economic goods. So there would be two sides of the same coin: either HIV/AIDS drives people underground and causes them to withdraw from the electoral process or it serves as a catalyst for infected and affected peoples to hold their representatives accountable for (lack of) service delivery.

We are supported by the outcomes of the Afrobarometer surveys which provide an analysis of citizen perceptions of state performances, in particular affecting health and AIDS. Through this instrument, we seek to understand whether AIDS is considered a national priority by Africans; the extent to which people experience HIV/AIDS at a personal level and their expectations in terms of government responsibility. While the Afrobarometer experts have done their own analysis of the findings, we attempt to go further in some respects to find other explanatory factors that cause Africans to express certain views. We therefore ask the question: does HIV/AIDS positively or negatively affect voter participation; if so, in what ways?

4. TERMINOLOGIES

In the course of discussing the spread of AIDS on the African continent, we shall constantly use words such as prevalence or incidence which might, in error, be confused by readers who are unfamiliar with the terminology. Prevalence refers to existing infections in the 15-49 age bands while incidence denotes new infections occurring in the same cohort each year. The 15-49 age cohort is the UNAIDS recommended measure to understand the extent of HIV in a population (or the percentage of persons aged between 15 and 49 who are infected with the virus (NAC, 2004)). This in effect means a 16% prevalence rate translates into 16% of 15-49-year olds being HIV-infected. It would not imply that 16% of the entire population in a country is infected, an error that AIDS experts constantly remind us in communicating HIV/AIDS national status (ibid).

5. CHOICE OF COUNTRIES

We selected the countries for this study on the basis of their electoral systems which needed to be compared in respect of their vulnerability to HIV/AIDS. In order for us to understand the dynamics of the disease, we needed to see whether countries with lower prevalence rates had a relatively low attrition rate among elected representatives, for instance. Southern African countries have exceedingly high levels of HIV in adult populations. Except for Mauritius, Seychelles and unexplored Angola and DRC, the other ten countries in the region carry a large caseload of HIV/AIDS cases (eight of them have adult prevalence of 15% or more).[20] The four other countries did not fit the bill for our purposes as the first two were islands and quite removed from mainland Africa. Angola and DRC were post-conflict nations with relatively weak institutions which would render it exceedingly difficult for us to gather information that would be reasonably comparable. We elected to include a West African state with a demonstrable record of early responses, a different history of colonisation and cultural experience, and a radically different religious make-up.

The seven countries eventually selected for this study were therefore Senegal, Botswana, Namibia, Malawi, Tanzania, South Africa and Zambia (The Botswana study was not completed in time to form part of this book.)

6. METHODOLOGY

In this study, the AIDS pandemic will be considered the independent variable while the electoral process is the dependent variable (Tredoux & Durrheim, 2002).[21]

The research has been structured around a standard methodology: Literature reviews of authoritative journals and studies; interviews with political party leaders, electoral officials, parliamentarians, election-based bodies; statistical analysis of epidemiological data, electoral data and Afrobarometer data; focus group discussions with PLWHAs and care-givers who are mainly registered or eligible voters; stakeholder meetings with cross-sectional participation from state and non-state actors.

Stakeholder meetings were held at the beginning of the research process where methodologies were discussed at national level and contributions made by other actors. These have been followed by post-research dissemination meetings with the same group of senior stakeholders where preliminary findings have been tested to the finalisation process. A number of dissemination/stakeholder meetings have also included official involvement from government ministers or speakers/deputy speakers of national parliaments, directors of electoral management bodies and presidents of leading political parties.

7. LIMITATIONS

We must, however, also state the difficulties encountered in pursuing this project. To begin with:

- Records on actual cause of death are not available due to confidentiality considerations. Researchers have had to draw inferences by analysing trends and age cohorts and determine whether they fit the AIDS mortality profiles;
- The available data on mortality among elected representatives is drawn from different periods of time in some respects. In countries such as Namibia and South Africa information prior to 1994 is scanty or non-existent;
- Not all countries have institutionalised citizen and voter registration systems; in cases where these exist, they will not always be directly compatible. This renders it extremely laborious for authorities to capture deaths and purge dead electors from the voters' rolls in time. Because of that, there is a high probability this investigation will not have unravelled the full extent to which voter registration systems have been compromised by AIDS, if at all;
- Some countries have not had a voters' register until recently or have changed the existing roll with every election, rendering longitudinal impact studies almost impossible to achieve as there is no guarantee of the accuracy of previous or current rolls. Also, such information is not directly comparable between countries because of the unique circumstances affecting each of them;
- As with all exploratory research, the project provides answers and also generates a myriad new questions. However, limited resources prevent the investigation of all perspectives that arise from this project.

CHAPTER TWO: MAKING SENSE OF DISPARITIES IN INFECTION RATES

1. INTRODUCTION

A global epidemic has consumed the world since the early 1980s when the HI virus was discovered, with Africa bearing the heaviest brunt. UNAIDS estimates that by December 2004 the epidemic had killed 20 million people and a total of between 35.9 and 44.3 million people worldwide were living with the virus. Of these 57% (25.4 million) are in Sub-Saharan Africa (UNAIDS/WHO: 2004; 2006).

HIV prevalence in Africa ranges from 0.7-9% in countries such as Senegal in West Africa; 1% in North Africa; to 15-30% in adult populations in most of southern Africa, the region most affected by the epidemic (CHGA; 2004: UNAIDS/WHO: 2005).

Figure 2.1: Population 2005

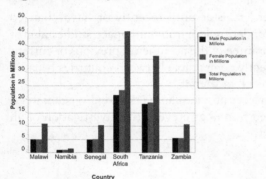

Source: WHO 2006, graph by Idasa

Leading health economists and social scientists have described AIDS as a "long wave" event (Barnett and Whiteside; 2002)[22]; one that will require long-term strategic planning and implementation to address its impact on current and future generations. HIV/AIDS is distinct from other epidemics and indeed other predominantly sexually transmitted diseases for several reasons:

• The symptoms are not immediately visible and can remain invisible for 10 years or more. This facilitates a silent diffusion through society via unprotected sex, poor medical facilities, intravenous drug use and Mother-To-Child Transmission (MTCT);

• Because it is a "catastrophe in slow motion", mostly transmitted through heterosexual intercourse, it comes with stigma and discrimination and therefore generates denial;

• Unlike other major killers such as tuberculosis, malaria or indeed other sexually transmitted infections (STIs), it has no cure;[23]

• It is unprecedented in terms of the human catastrophe it has caused;

• It is the first disease to be labelled a global security threat by the United Nations Security Council, and the first to command a discussion by the entire Security Council (Hunter: 2003).

Since its manifestation, life expectancy in southern Africa has declined from 60 years to below 40 years in the most affected countries, particularly in the sub-region defined by the Southern African Development Community (SADC), which constitutes Angola, Botswana, the Democratic Republic of Congo (DRC), Lesotho, Mauritius, Malawi, Mozambique, Namibia, Seychelles, South Africa, Swaziland, Tanzania, Zambia and Zimbabwe.

Figure 2.2: HIV/AIDS prevalence 2005

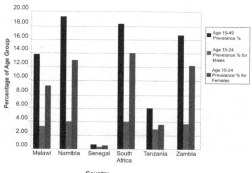

Source: WHO 2006; graph by Idasa

Figure 2.3: Adult mortality per 1 000 (2004)

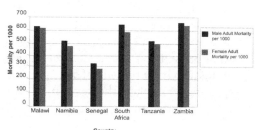

Source: WHO 2006

Data from 2006 suggest the SADC hosts less than 2% of the global population,[24] but by many accounts has the highest concentration of HIV in the world, with approximately 39% or 14.9 million of the 38.6 million people living with HIV (at the end of 2006). The region carries the additional burden of 41% of children orphaned by AIDS.[25]

Due to the decimation of working age populations, food security and nutrition have been under threat. Agriculture, the mainstay of the majority of the people in the region, is already experiencing the impact of HIV/AIDS. The Food and Agricultural Organisation (FAO) estimates that more than seven million workers have been lost due to HIV/AIDS in the Sub-Saharan region, with agriculture experiencing the severest impact. The SADC also acknowledges the effect on business in the sub-region as productivity declines due to absenteeism and deaths amongst workers and profit margins are compromised as spending on sickness and death benefits rises (SADC: 2003).

Strategic institutions such as government departments are enduring a growing skills gap and need to attract foreign labour. AIDS-related illnesses are also affecting recruitment and training amongst the armed forces as relatively large numbers of eligible candidates are eliminated while serving officers are left out of international training programmes due to their HIV status (UNAIDS: 2006).

Despite AIDS, during the mid to late 1990s, population growth rates in the SADC increased, with some countries reporting growth rates of 3.5% per annum. Experts attributed the growth rates to a fall in infant mortality rates and the sustenance of high fertility levels in the SADC which increased from 4.9 in 1990 to 5.1 in 1997. This picture had changed by the dawn of the millennium.

Mortality amongst adults in several countries has since trebled. The trends show increases in infant mortality as more children became infected. Generally, mortality profiles in the region, according to some experts, have become reminiscent of the 1950s (SADC: 2003)[26].

The SADC predicts that the unprecedented demographic effects of the HIV epidemic will have dire implications for the social and economic development of the region:

Figure 2.4: Average life expectancy (2004)

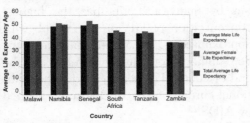

Source: WHO 2006

• The overall population growth is predicted to be lower than it would have been without HIV/AIDS;
• Poverty will increase amongst the populations of the region unless significant response mechanism are deployed;
• The ILO predicts that by 2010 the labour force in countries with the highest rates will have labour forces 20% smaller than they would have had under conditions of no-AIDS (ibid).

2. WHY IS THE SADC MOST AFFECTED BY HIV/AIDS?

Why is the SADC region the most affected by HIV/AIDS on the continent? Why are infection levels so much lower in western and northern Africa? While a detailed scientific explanation of these phenomena is beyond the expertise of this study, we can briefly examine some of the key reasons advanced over time by experts from various disciplines.

The reasons posited constitute a combination of pre-existing social, cultural, legal, economic and political conditions which were thought to have provided fertile ground for the spread of HIV.[27] Initial arguments attempting to explain the severity of the SADC AIDS epidemic were at best speculative. Some of the inter-linking factors that are today discussed are as follows:[28]

• High levels of gender-based violence and particularly sexual violence and rape of women and children;
• Low HIV risk perception;
• Pervasiveness of transactional and transgenerational sex among young people, especially young women;[29]
• The HI Virus (type 1) found in the SADC region is more virulent than the type 2 found in West Africa;[30]
• Social, cultural and legal practices that place women in an unequal position in society and thus increases their exposure to HIV/AIDS;[31]
• High mobility and varied patterns of migration, some of which is specifically linked to employment and was particularly central to the economic and political history of the region;
• High levels of politically-motivated conflict and violence for at least the last 20 years in individual countries within the region, including internal displacements;[32]
• High levels of multiple and concurrent sexual partnerships by men and women with insufficient consistent, correct condom use, combined with low levels of male circumcision are the key drivers of the epidemic in the sub-region.[33]

Some of the arguments may not have general validity and will therefore not explain the disparities in infection rates between southern and western Africa, mainly because the studies appear to be concentrated in the SADC region.

In relation to human mobility, Crush et al (2006) explain that the incidence of HIV in Sub-Saharan Africa has been found to be higher near roads where people profess to have personal migration experience or have migrants for sexual partners. Infection rates amongst migrants in western and southern Africa have also been found to be comparatively higher than in the general population. Truck drivers, probably the most studied group of all, have been the hardest hit. One of the most cited forms of human mobility, cross-border migration, could also occur because people with AIDS-related illnesses travel to neighbouring countries seeking better medical care. Others will migrate to seek higher paying jobs that can help support their families, some of whom may be stricken by AIDS. The need to replace workers who have died from AIDS could force governments to import skilled labour. Illegal immigrants, refugees and Internally Displaced Persons (IDPs) will be extremely vulnerable to HIV/AIDS and may come in contact with local populations or be abused by them.[34]

> The need to replace workers who have died from AIDS could force governments to import skilled labour.

The argument for conflict (leading to displacement) as a vector for the spread of HIV and as an explanation for higher prevalence rates in SADC as opposed to western Africa is still weak and largely lacking in empirical evidence. Information from the UN suggests that IDPs still constitute a problem in the SADC region despite the resolution of conflict. But there is a lack of data to substantiate these assertions. The causes of displacement are diverse but inter-related: displacement is discussed as a defining feature of colonialism, whose effects have not been fully addressed. Displacement was also a distinct objective of South Africa under the apartheid regime. While armed conflict is highlighted as a major cause of displacement in the post-colonial era (wars in Angola, the DRC and Mozambique stand out), there appear to be other factors that contribute significantly to mass movement of people in the SADC region. Human rights violations, political violence and urban renewal operations such as Zimbabwe's Operation Murambatsvina (drive out filth) are a case in point. Natural disasters such as droughts, cyclones, floods and volcanic eruptions also prompt sudden movements of people to escape the peril of the fallout.[35]

The parallels with West Africa are somewhat different if conflict is defined to mean armed conflict. Most of West Africa was characterised by political violence and executions soon after the toppling of civilian post-independence governments by military officers in the 1960s and 70s. The era of the military regimes spanned more than two decades. In addition, there were several countries at a time torn by full-scale armed conflicts (civil wars) covering an entire country in most instances. West African trouble spots such as Liberia, Sierra Leone, Ivory Coast and Guinea-Bissau have experienced civil war over long periods at a time punctuated by gross abuse of human rights.

In trying to quell it, the Economic Community of West African States (ECOWAS), the equivalent of the SADC in West Africa, has fought fire with fire: military tactics have been employed to stamp out wars, led by Nigeria.[36] Even with this background, no authoritative studies have established strong correlations between HIV/AIDS and conflict.[37]

Perhaps in understanding the SADC AIDS conundrum, we should critically consider the advent of peace as a facilitator of unprecedented levels of interaction between the sub-region's peoples, for better or for worse. UNDP's 2000 SADC Human Development Report underlines the fact that relative peace and stability and improved road and rail infrastructure have facilitated more effective movement of people and goods.

Eleven inter-state highways and rail systems criss-cross at least 12 countries of the region, leading to 15 ports located at the Indian and Atlantic oceans. Improved infrastructure and arteries between member states and a relaxation of visa requirements in some respects have all aided the movement of the SADC region's peoples. We may summarise the incentives for movements as such:

- Improved transport (including cheaper flights between states, since the introduction of budget airlines);
- Growth of communication systems disseminates images of places of opportunity (employment, trade, tourism etc.);
- Opening up of once-closed borders like Namibia and South Africa;
- Increasing international trade and commerce (formal and informal) and increasing free trade;
- Better educational opportunities in neighbouring states.[38]

Migration, therefore, could be categorised as involuntary induced by destabilisation or voluntary which connotes movement of people for professional or economic reasons such as truck drivers, seafarers, agricultural workers, students, teachers, sex workers, traders, members of the armed forces and mine workers.

In May 2006, further attempts were made by experts to explain the difference in infection levels between southern and western Africa. A "think tank" held in Lesotho by the SADC and UNAIDS explained the higher levels of infection in southern Africa thus: "high levels of multiple and concurrent sexual partnerships by men and women with insufficient consistent, correct condom use, combined with low levels of male circumcision are the key drivers of the epidemic in the sub-region."(Halperin and Epstein: 2006). The meeting recommended as the two major strategies national circumcision campaigns and the need for a significant reduction in multiple partnerships for men and women.

Figure 2.5: AIDS deaths (2002)

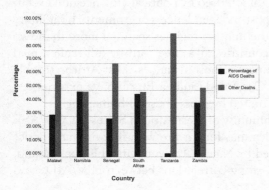

Daniel Halperin and Helen Epstein (2006) elucidate that there is now conclusive evidence of an epidemiological and biological nature confirming the strong correlation between male circumcision and HIV which apparently explains "much of the five-fold difference in HIV rates between southern and western Africa". They caution however that in Asia and Europe, where circumcision is also uncommon, the HIV prevalence rates remain inexplicably and comparatively much, much lower. The differences in HIV infection rates based on circumcision or lack of it have not yet been studied outside of Africa.

The immediate controversial assertion would be that southern Africans or Sub-Saharan Africans are more sexually liberal than their Arabic, North African neighbours or their European or American counterparts. However, recent demographic and health surveys suggest that on average African men typically do not have more sexual partners than elsewhere. The WHO's comparative study in the 1990s revealed that men in Thailand and Rio de Janeiro in Brazil were more likely to report five or more casual sexual partners in the previous year than were men in Tanzania, Kenya, Lesotho or Zambia. The number of women who reported having five or more partners a year was even lower.

> "Men and women in Africa report roughly similar, if not fewer, numbers of lifetime partners than do heterosexuals in many western countries," (Halperin and Epstein; 2006).

Epidemiologists have however observed that Africans of both sexes usually have more than one concurrent partnership that can overlap for months or years and cite WHO studies which show that 18%, 22% and 55% of men in Tanzania, Lusaka and Lesotho respectively reported entertaining two or more regular, year-long, sexual partnerships during the previous year. Conversely, only 3% of men in Thailand and 2% in Sri Lanka reported similar profiles (ibid).

Therefore the distinctive feature, according to Halperin and Epstein, is that the pattern of concurrent partnerships which characterises (southern) Africa is markedly different from that of serial monogamy that is prevalent in the west.[39]

3. SENEGAL

Arguments that point to denial, which punctuated the early years of AIDS, as a key factor that compromised an early SADC response will also hold their own. Senegal and Uganda are credited for early mobilisation and strategic thinking on handling the advent of HIV/AIDS.

While southern Africa seems to project abuse of women and unregulated sex work, Cheikh Ibrahima Niang's[40] analysis of power structures reveals a deep appreciation of women's political power in the pre-colonial societies of West Africa which still forms the bedrock of influence today. Current approaches to dealing with HIV/AIDS draw upon the local culture to develop responses and strategies which give the local communities a sense of historical and cultural continuity and expression, with women constituting a source of social mobilisation, he argues.

Unlike the SADC states, Senegal prior to the emergence of AIDS had also set up a number of political, legal and social arrangements aiming at the regulation of sex work, policies for blood transfusion safety, the management of sexually transmitted diseases, the reform of the health system, and support to women and youth movements.

With an institutional and response framework already in place, the government of Senegal was able to swiftly operationalise national multi-disciplinary approaches to deal with the epidemic, led by its Prime Minister. Niang argues that the response embraced principles of devolution, decentralisation, multi-sector planning, respect for equity and the rights of People Living With HIV/AIDS (PLWHAs), and continuous evaluation against the guiding principles of UNAIDS. The Senegalese leadership was able to mobilise actors across all spectrums, including respected religious leaders, to galvanise their communities. The success story is corroborated by other authorities who itemise the strong points as: early political engagement; a strong civil society response; and one of the earliest national initiatives for antiretroviral therapy (ART) access. Hence, funds from the Global Fund to Fight AIDS, TB and Malaria and the World Bank's Multi-country HIV/AIDS Programme for Africa (MAP) bolstered pre-existing, strong national programmatic and financial commitments.[41] The response does have its critics though. The international HIV/AIDS Alliance asserts that the scaling-up of the Senegalese strategy lacked clear vision and strategy and was found wanting in terms of its failure to target orphans and vulnerable children and other disadvantaged populations; it questions whether respect for the rights and dignity of PLWHAs was indeed extended as claimed; and highlights the sense that access to HIV testing and ARV treatment remained limited.[42]

> The Senegalese leadership was able to mobilise actors across all spectrums to galvanise their communities.

The role of religion as an additional neutralising instrument might also be appreciated in curbing what might be described as deviant behaviour. Certainly, it appears no coincidence that mainland Tanzania has a much higher HIV-prevalence rate (at 7% in 2004) than the predominantly Islamic island of Zanzibar (less than 1% prevalence and 4.7% incidence in 2004; UNAIDS; 2005), despite regular interaction between inhabitants of both land masses and with tourists. Senegal watchers have cited religion as an important factor, provided some flexibility is exercised in terms of how the moral code is applied. The involvement of Islamic and Christian protective norms, such as abstinence before marriage, fidelity and care of those affected early on are strong considerations in the success of the Senegalese response. Senegal, despite the prevalence of religion, was also apparently able to promote the use of condoms through church elders. Those who could not abstain were advised to use condoms. The dialogical culture in Senegal is highlighted as one of the cardinal approaches that led to effective networking amongst various interests to subvert AIDS.[43]

4. SADC IN PERSPECTIVE: POLITICAL, ECONOMIC INTEGRATION IN THE AGE OF HIV/AIDS

It is a strange paradox in some ways that the SADC, a regional body that has shown so much promise in terms of democratisation, integration and problem-solving, is the one saddled with a crisis that seems from time to time to defy any efforts at reversal.

With a population of 240 million people and endowed with mineral wealth ranging from oil, natural gas, copper, diamonds, cobalt, to phosphates and uranium, this region of Africa is also blessed with incredible hydroelectric potential in shared water courses.[44]

It is the relatively more stable part of the Sub-Saharan continent and is distinctive in the way it led the democratisation process through generally acceptable electoral processes in the 1990s. Guided by a common framework of principles and developmental goals, the SADC seeks to build common political and economic institutions to be able to compete in a highly globalised world market. It forms part of the vision of the Organisation of African Unity (OAU) the forerunner of the African Union (AU), to develop Regional Economic Communities (RECs) as building blocks for an integrated continent. Other RECs include ECOWAS, the Economic Community of Central African States (ECCAS) and the Arab Maghreb Union (AMU). To its credit, the SADC has managed its shared resources through a set of protocols and institutions that play critical distributive and allocative functions and avert potential conflict over resources and other contentious matters.

The events that led to the formation of the SADC began in 1970 with the idea of a military alliance of three countries – Botswana, Tanzania and Zambia – called the Frontline States (FLS). The alliance was created to fight for the liberation of territories under white minority rule; i.e. Angola, Mozambique, South West Africa (now Namibia), Rhodesia (now Zimbabwe) and South Africa with the aim of realising fundamental freedoms for all peoples. It became formally operational in 1975 with Mozambique and Angola, now independent, becoming the fourth and fifth members of the FLS respectively. In 1979, with Rhodesia on the verge of liberation, the FLS was transformed into the Southern African Development Co-ordinating Conference (SADCC) embracing the newly liberated territories. The SADCC was officially launched in 1980 in Lusaka, Zambia with the focus on economic cooperation and installing majority rule in South Africa and Namibia, the last bastions of apartheid.[45]

With the emergence of globalisation, the SADCC was reconstituted in 1992 and renamed the Southern African Development Community (SADC). Namibia and South Africa became its newest members. The SADC's founding treaty was based on deeper economic integration and democracy.[46] Its formation was in response to envisaged threats to human development in the sub-region and the need to develop strategies to avert these. Some of these were:

• The need to create mechanisms to address civil wars within member states;

• The limited size of the economies, which made countries individually unattractive to investment and integration therefore a natural choice if the region was to remain competitive in a globalised environment;

• The relatively small population size of most SADC countries meant the per capita cost of providing infrastructure was high but could be reduced if countries cooperated in developing new infrastructure;

• Lastly, the emergence of HIV/AIDS, TB, malaria and other infectious diseases across borders called for collaboration at all levels between nations.[47]

Despite making headway in areas such as environmental management, transport, energy, peace and security, the SADC was, through its first decade of existence, unable to satisfy the general measure of human progress in the Human Development Index (HDI), which is composed of three elements of human development: longevity, education level and living standards.

The Development Policy Research Unit (DPRU) of the University of Cape Town explains that measuring HDI relies on proxy indicators. For instance, longevity is proxied by life expectancy, education by levels of enrolment and adult literacy rates and living standards by income. The DPRU indicates further that the average HDI value for the SADC region in 1998 was 0.538, which was considered to be a medium human development level (The value of the human development categories range from 0.800-1.000 (high); to 0.500 to 0.799 (medium) and 0.000-0.499 (low).

Seychelles, with a HDI value of 0.808, Mauritius with 0.782 and South Africa with 0.718 had the highest levels of human progress in the region, while Mozambique (0.350), Malawi (0.393) and Angola (0.419) had the lowest. The studies show that the value of SADC-specific HDI declined 5.3% between 1995 and 1998, indicating relatively slow progress toward improved living standards, education levels and longevity. The sharpest declines were in the DRC (-0.065), South Africa (-0.040) and Angola (-0.029).[48] The SADC attributes the negative trends in HDI mainly to HIV/AIDS (SADC; 2003).

Table 2.1: SADC human development categories (based on HDI values)	
High human development category	Seychelles
Medium human development category	Mauritius, South Africa, Swaziland, Namibia, Botswana, Lesotho and Zimbabwe
Low human development category	DRC, Zambia, Tanzania, Angola, Malawi and Mozambique
Source: DPRU Policy Briefs No. 01/p13, May 2001.	

The gross combined enrolment ratio at primary, secondary and tertiary levels rose between 1980 and 1995 from 38% to 51%. It, however, dipped to 51.14% in 1998. The adult literacy rate for the SADC increased from 48% in 1970 to 71% in 1995. The levels dropped to 67.32% in 1998. Adult literacy rates were highest in Angola, Mozambique and Malawi (58%, 57.7 % and 41% respectively).

Gross Domestic Product (GDP) the element in the HDI that measures living standards showed that the Seychelles (10 600), Mauritius (8 312) and South Africa (8 488), were the highest earners while Zambia (719), Malawi (523) and Tanzania (480) were the lowest.

The Regional Indicative Strategic Development Plan (RISDP), a 15-year regional integration development framework launched in 2004, now targets an annual economic growth rate of at least 7%, which is believed to be necessary to halve the proportion of people living in poverty by 2015.[49] The RISDP and Strategic Indicative Plan for the Organ on Politics, Defence and Security Cooperation (SIPO) represent more recent efforts by SADC to achieve its integration aims while collectively tackling its major challenges of infrastructural development, poverty reduction and combating disease (including AIDS), among other things.

4.1 SADC STRATEGIC FRAMEWORK 2000-2004

Confronted with the urgent need to integrate and compete in the global market and at the same time mitigate the impact of AIDS, SADC developed its first major response framework on HIV/AIDS for the period 2000-2004, which facilitated a number of processes including defining and promoting best practices, programme delivery, research and policy, capacity building and development of standards. However, the regional response could not adequately operationalise a multisector approach as only a limited number of its 21 sectors based in 14 countries in reality implemented any form of strategy.

The plan also lacked in-depth knowledge of the non-health impacts of HIV/AIDS. This limited scope was demonstrated by the body's inclination toward charging the responsibility for managing AIDS affairs to the SADC Health Sector Coordinating Unit (SADC-HSCU). Some other key shortcomings of the framework, as identified by a technical review of the plan in 2002, included:

- Failure to include the food security and finance sectors in the plan, despite being central to the region's development;
- Although some success was noted in the development of the SADC Code of Conduct on HIV/AIDS and employment, mechanisms for monitoring among member states were not put in place, hence discrimination against PLWHAs remained unchecked at national levels;
- The development of the strategic plan had not been supported by the necessary resources to effect implementation;
- The plan lacked the skills and capacity to mainstream HIV/AIDS. Most SADC sectors were saddled with other functions and could not cope with an additional task (SADC: 2003).

4.2 THE NEW SADC STRATEGIC FRAMEWORK AND PLAN OF ACTION, 2003-2007

In the new vision of 2003-2007, the SADC evidently broadened its understanding of the epidemic's impacts and its technical teams interacted more with new research and issues emerging from civil society and the private sector. The revised strategy was also aided in part by a restructuring exercise that collapsed the multiple sectors into technical clusters housed in one secretariat in Gaborone, Botswana.

SADC sectors dealing with a wide range of development issues, including health, environment, mining, trade, investment and tourism,[50] underwent a major restructuring exercise to concentrate its operations under the secretariat in Gaborone. Four directorates were established to lead all its functions. An HIV/AIDS unit was also established at the secretariat, within the Department of Strategic Planning, Gender and Policy Harmonisation. Each of the four directorates at SADC was assigned an HIV/AIDS specialist who would report to the unit head and who would in turn report to the chief director.

SADC national committees were recommended to lead activities at national levels, which included coordinating and mobilising the national consensus on regional responses, implementation and monitoring. The National AIDS Councils would be the secretariat to the national technical committees on AIDS-related matters. The SADC framework would also complement national and regional efforts at resource mobilisation.

Operational budgets were allocated to the Department of Strategic Planning, Gender and Policy Harmonisation, the Directorate for Social and Human Development and Special Programmes, the Directorate for Trade, Industry, Finance and Investment, the Directorate for Infrastructure and Services, the Directorate of Food, Agriculture and Natural Resources, and the Organ on Politics, Defence and Security. The plan, devised by a group of consultants, identified five key cross-cutting areas in which to direct the efforts of its streamlined secretariat and directorates:

- Human capital: the SADC needed to recognise that the depletion of human capital would have consequences for social, economic and political activity;
- Public goods: the SADC's activities depended on the effectiveness of public administration and the supply of goods, and therefore strategies for addressing the erosion of state capacity were required;
- Intersectoral relationships: SADC policies needed to address interlinkages between the political, economic and social aspects of the pandemic to be effective;
- Investment strategies: the SADC needed to ensure that investments in different programme areas were coordinated and were supportive of each other in the response to the pandemic. The application of labour-saving technology could compensate for the losses in human capital for instance in the agriculture sector.
- Integrating gender: SADC policies needed to mainstream gender matters, delving deeper into the power and social relations between men and women. Women were the more prolific group in agriculture labour in the region; they not only played a bigger role in raising children and passing on life skills but were also more generally central to the economy. They, regrettably, are also the group that is disproportionately affected by the HIV/AIDS pandemic.

SADC's vision for 2003-2007 hence aimed to achieve the following:

- To reduce the incidence of new infections among the most vulnerable groups within the SADC;
- To mitigate the socio-economic impact of HIV/AIDS;
- To review, develop and harmonise policies and legislation relating to HIV prevention, care and support, and treatment within the SADC;
- To mobilise and coordinate resources for a multi-sectoral response to HIV/AIDS in the SADC region.

This time the regional body also emphasised the need for harmonisation,[51] monitoring the implementation of the SADC framework in addition to keeping tabs on member states' adherence to regional, continental and global commitments. Lastly, greater emphasis was laid on ensuring that gender was mainstreamed (SADC: 2003).

It is important to state that although the regional response came much later, member states of the SADC had operationalised their national responses targeting HIV prevention, care and support, and the mitigation of the socio-economic impact of HIV/AIDS since the mid-1980s. Their primary reference point was the WHO's Global Programme on AIDS assisted by other multilateral and bilateral donors. The early national responses were essentially health-focused and it was not until the 1990s that the multi-sector approach was adopted and mechanisms developed. Meanwhile, pressure for increased investment in health began to grow from lobby groups and activists across the globe. African governments were not spared.

4.3 AIDS RESOURCE FLOWS

While there has been increased donor funding flows to AIDS interventions and African governments have shown a measure of political commitment, these developments are still to be translated into action through adequate resource allocation. The last two to five years have seen various countries introduce programmes to provide free ART in the public sector, financed through their own country and/or foreign sources. Despite the fact that governments have increased nominal allocations towards HIV/AIDS, empirical evidence has shown that over the years, public resources allocated to health have been decreasing owing to over-reliance on donor aid. Dependency on donor funds raises concerns about the sustainability of massive treatment programmes over decades.[52]

Figure 2.6: Development aid for HIV/AIDS: How much is going to which countries?

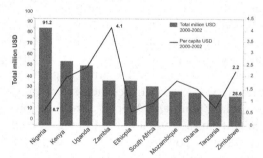

Source: OECD/UNAIDS special study: Aid Activities in Support of HIV/AIDS Control for 2000-2002

Even countries with enough domestic resources to shore up large-scale AIDS prevention, treatment and care interventions, such as South Africa, have experienced problems of limited absorptive capacity which affects the overall execution of its programme. Differences in provinces' readiness, capacity and political will are leading to significantly varied results in the ARV rollout, with the worst-performing provinces covering only 10% of those newly in need of care (Ndhlovu & Daswa 2006:2). Specifically, readiness and capacity are often a function of visionary leadership and strong managerial skills (De Renzio, 2004:5).

Most governments have failed to adhere to the Abuja Declaration (2001) which stipulates that they allocate 15% of their national budgets to the health sector. But their ambitions to adhere to international norms do not appear diminished.

SADC member states, like other African countries, have in this regard linked their strategies to the Millennium Development Goals (MDGs). But given the myriad challenges facing the sub-region and Africa in general, and the relatively limited resources available, there is grave doubt whether some of the goals will be achieved. In the context of AIDS, we may draw some encouragement from the availability of treatment – albeit limited – and increased investments in health (and dutifully consider treatment as a moderating variable). However, we must also be mindful that socioeconomic analysis warns of the monumental task required to meet global developmental targets.

In fact recent reports indicate that the extent of HIV/AIDS is such that southern Africa is unlikely to meet the Millennium Development Goal 6: halving and reversing the spread of HIV/AIDS (malaria and other diseases) by 2015. Treatment not withstanding, indications thus far also suggest that it will be extremely ambitious to expect universal access to anti-retroviral drugs (ARVs) by 2015. And although the number of people on ART in low- and middle-income countries almost doubled in 2005 from 720 000 to 1.3 million, new infections far outstripped this figure at 4.9 million in the same year (UN General Assembly 16th session, 2006).[53]

Tuberculosis-related deaths have soared since 1990 and the prevalence rates are still in the double digits in most countries. Despite some gains in orphan education, the AIDS factor is complicated further by the region's anticipated failure to meet the Millennium Development Goal 1: redress extreme poverty and hunger. Food insecurity and child malnutrition are likely to remain relentless adversaries for the foreseeable future. Similarly, maternal health is compromised by the relatively high mortality rate among mothers, which is being attributed mainly to HIV/AIDS.

There is more hope that Africa may meet its targets in some areas demanding gender equality such as access to education, but we are still a long way from achieving parity in employment.[54] The situation of orphans continues to deteriorate with southern Africa, again, bearing the brunt: 13 million orphans will need support as they strive to reach adulthood. Further, people with HIV/AIDS-related diseases continue to occupy more than half of all hospital beds in the high-prevalence countries of Sub-Saharan Africa, straining available services beyond capacity in most instances. Health professionals are at risk of infection due to inadequate infection control measures; they are also poorly paid and have been leaving Africa in droves for lucrative opportunities in western countries (ibid). Africans, especially southern Africans, are therefore caught in a complex reinforcing vortex of disease, poverty, food insecurity, poor infrastructure and low literacy rates, among other things, all of which lead to a massive governance challenge (UNAIDS; 2006).

Figure 2.7: Are African states meeting the Abuja declaration?

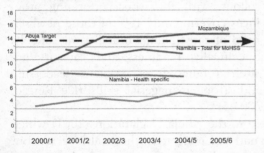

Source: Idasa, Funding the Fight, Budgeting for HIV/ AIDS in developing countries, 2004 page 235.

This suggests that it has taken us well over 20 years to begin to realise that AIDS is a much larger epidemic than simply a health crisis affecting only one sector or a handful of countries. Years of formulating and reformulating strategies have brought us to a point where notions of governance and human security are beginning to play their part in the analysis of the pandemic's trajectory and impacts and hopefully are starting to inform our future responses.

To fully appreciate this discussion, we must critically interrogate the related concepts of governance and democratic governance and how they are being related to HIV/AIDS in current academic discourse. We shall steer the discourse to the role the electoral process plays in democratic governance and how it is affected by the pandemic.

CHAPTER THREE:
HIV/AIDS AND DEMOCRATIC GOVERNANCE

1. DEFINING GOVERNANCE

It is critical to emphasise that the relationship between HIV/AIDS and governance is highly complex and calls for focus in terms of how we interrogate the related issues. Extreme caution has to be exercised not to get caught up in the often confusing discourse on governance and the more normative notion of democratic governance. There is a plethora of literature that indicates that these concepts lack global consensus on their constituent elements. Hyden, Court and Mease (2004: 12) are instructive in this regard: "despite the recent popularity of governance at both practical and theoretical levels, the concept continues to mean different things to different people."

In several bodies of literature, governance as a tool is understood to facilitate a strategic developmental interaction between state and non-state actors in the management of the political, economic and social affairs of a country.[55] Much of today's understanding of the term revolves around the thought that governance is a non-hierarchical form of coordinating policy-making.

Mayntz (2003) traces the modern theory of political governance back to post-World War II when conflict-wary governments sought to steer their nations to result-defined social and economic goals. Over the decades the use of terms such as coordination, network and decentralisation punctuated theoretical discussions on governance. The concept grew in significance in international discourse in the 1980s promoted by the World Bank and other multilateral donors. African scholars assert that the continent interrogated these concepts at about the same time.

The Khartoum Declaration of 1988, for instance, highlighted the promotion of human development, restoration of basic human rights and freedoms, overcoming political instability and intolerance and decentralisation of power (UNDP 2000). The African Charter for Popular Participation and Transformation crafted at Arusha, Tanzania in 1990 went further to emphasise accountability of leadership, press freedom and economic justice as key elements of governance.

There is some consonance in the manner in which the UNDP, the AU, the IMF and the World Bank articulate governance as a concept, each agreeing that it can be broken into different domains, all of which have policy import. These broadly encompass political, economic and social domains. The acceptance of human rights as core elements of governance by the World Bank albeit under considerable pressure from bilateral donors has moved the major international players to some common ground on the definition of the concept and its indicators in this regard (Hyden et al: 2004).

However, Hyden, Court and Mease (2004) argue that international development agencies have tended to avoid the political character of governance in their indicators because their official terms of reference for a long time barred them from working with political entities. This disconnection caused the political feature of governance "to lose its distinction in relation to the economy". More recently, there has been a convergence of opinion on political governance as the arena in which policy is formulated. UNDP elaborates: not only does political governance revolve around conditioning the quality of governance more generally, it has important constituent elements including basic political rights, freedom of expression, supremacy of the rule of law, broad participation of citizens in local governance and community forums and competitive, free and fair elections[56] (UNDP 2000), all of which facilitate the involvement of non-state actors in policy processes.

It is certain that the early attempts at analysing governance overlooked the African context: African scholars will agree that policies on the continent are usually externally defined by multilateral institutions and should not therefore see themselves as "conditioning" economic governance through politics based on their own actions only.

In fact, in later publications, the UNDP undertakes to include corporate and global governance as overriding phenomena which affect the way national governments determine their priorities. It asserts that local decisions are not always the result of national government actions but come under considerable influence from global capital. In most cases national entities, including governments, must negotiate with transnational companies and multilateral and bilateral partners to enable the allocative and distributive functions of their political, economic and social policies to take root.

> **It is certain that the early attempts at analysing governance overlooked the African context.**

Economic governance, in this sense, involves decision-making processes that affect a country's economic activities and its relationship with other economies. Economic governance also includes other key players such as trade unions, chambers of commerce, reserve banks and farming communities, the International Monetary Fund (IMF) and the World Bank (UNDP; 2000; p. 12). It is this aspect of governance that should ensure that access to the basic necessities of life, such as education, food security, welfare and health, i.e. all goals of human development, is delivered.

Finally, administrative governance is identified as the arena in which rules are implemented. There are four important observations to be made from these definitions:

- Governance can be divided into distinct domains; political, economic, administrative and corporate/global contexts all of which buttress human development;
- Governance is underpinned by a set of principles or values, which may be informed by internationally defined human rights instruments, and/or in the case of many developing states, indicators imposed by multilateral and bilateral agencies;
- Governance represents a horizontal form of policy interaction characterised by different modes of coordinating individual actions, or basic forms of social order;
- Governance is broader than government, as it embraces non-state actors in policy processes that may lead to sustainable human development.

1.1 "GOOD" OR DEMOCRATIC GOVERNANCE

While there has not been much disagreement on the characteristics of governance, there was, for a long time, less consensus on what constituted "good governance" a post-cold war era concept that responded to the demands of global multilateral institutions or their beneficiaries. This post-cold war discourse was penned on political conditionalities which rewarded democratising regimes with loans and development aid and punished authoritarian and neo-patrimonial regimes with economic sanctions (UNDP: 2000). Conditionalities included the liberalisation of the political spectrum, accountability, transparency and observance of the rule of law.

Hyden et al. (2004: 2) observes that international organisations have made stronger attempts to reach consensus on what constitutes "good" governance largely based on an array of measures reflecting western historical experiences of democracy, and impliedly takes no account of Africa's own interpretations of the concepts.

To understand how this plays out in the discourse on democratisation in Africa we turn to respected intellectual Moletsi Mbeki, who emphasises that in fact Africa's much celebrated wave of democratisation in the 1990s had significant external interventions and was not primarily a result of pro-democracy actions by local organisations.[57] Mbeki's arguments reinforce undercurrents from within African academia and activism that posit that the model of democracy adopted by African countries is an imposition by multilateral agencies through the complex web of conditionalities that demand liberal market environments conducive to economic colonisation.

1.2 DEMOCRATIC GOVERNANCE IN AFRICA IN THE FACE OF HIV/AIDS

Supporters of western democracy boast that the system has an unequalled record as the most accomplished form of governance in which political and socio-economic human rights are respected and conflicts resolved peacefully (NIMD: 2004). It is argued that democracies facilitate broad avenues for redress, contestation, expression and participation and hence present the best option for dealing with HIV/AIDS, taking into account the political, social and economic rights of those living with the disease.

Proponents and critics alike will however converge on one line of argument: democracies appear to be more difficult to consolidate in periods of poor economic performance, poverty and disease. Also, decision-making of an emergency nature may sometimes be stalled by uncompromising opposition standpoints in the legislature. Certainly decisions relating to an epidemic such as HIV/AIDS might also suffer, depending on the leverage the party in power has (Strand, Matlosa, Strode and Chirambo; 2005). It would also be unrealistic to assume that the rules in a democracy are applied fairly to poor people, women or minorities. Often this imbalance will arise as resources and opportunities are not always equitably allocated in areas which would be broadly empowering for the disadvantaged, leading to the unintended consequences of illiteracy, poverty and so on.

Democracies can also be unsettled by power alternations. The highly unstable situation in Malawi for example provides some invaluable lessons on the vulnerability of democracy in this regard. Since the election of the current president, Dr Bingu Wa Mutharika, in 2004 by a slender margin, his tenure has been undermined by incessant efforts by the opposition to impeach him. Although he has survived most attempts and appears to be gaining in popularity generally, long drawn out deliberations on impeachment for a long time diverted attention from key issues, such as debt cancellation and AIDS relief.

> **The situation in Malawi provides some invaluable lessons on the vulnerability of democracy.**

Authoritarian regimes or nominally democratic states have tended to act more swiftly and decisively against HIV/AIDS. Uganda, Thailand, Cuba and the North African states are some of those that can boast of low prevalence or a significantly reduced level of current and new infections. The trouble with authoritarianism arises when the government in power decides to ignore HIV/AIDS or any other matter of public policy concern: there may be no alternative avenues to challenge such an administration. Its weaknesses notwithstanding, therefore, we have to accept in the end that democracy in its many variants remains the dominant system of governance in the world today.

In this regard, the UNDP has added an even sharper normative edge to the concept of good governance by applying (western inspired) democratic values more critically. Good governance is now equated with democratic governance; embracing such institutions as freedom of expression and association, vibrant civil societies, gender equity and equality, rule of law, fundamental human rights, media freedom and free and fair elections.

2. DEMOCRATIC GOVERNANCE PRINCIPLES IN THE CONTEXT OF HIV/AIDS

Drawing on the plethora of literature and Idasa's own experiences of democracy, this book embraces, with some reservations, the global interpretation of "good" or democratic governance in the context of HIV/AIDS as constructed by the UNDP. The constituent elements of democratic governance in this regard, with Idasa's embellishments, will be defined by the following principles:

UNDP 1: *People's human rights and fundamental freedoms are respected, allowing them to live with dignity.*

Idasa 1: Idasa's interpretation and working definition of democracy encompasses a commitment to social justice that is captured in our mission statement; democratic transition must be accompanied by a substantive improvement in the material conditions in which people live and work. In relation to public health, a balance must be struck between respecting the rights of those who are infected as well as the rights of those who are not. The individual's rights to privacy about their HIV status and treatment for AIDS are as fundamental as their right to protection from

HIV. Any political intervention that imposes on any of these rights must be legiti-mised through public deliberation and due legal process.

UNDP 2: People have a say in decisions that affect their lives.

Idasa 2: Participation – or "active citizenship" as it is called in Idasa's mission state-ment – is fundamental to a modern, working democracy. The right to access to information and to participative processes at all the key moments in the policy- and law-making cycle – such as the annual budget process – are critical levers to social upliftment. Only by creating political space for poor people to have their voices heard will institutions of governance be responsive to the needs and interests of the most vulnerable members of society. Thus, policies on HIV/AIDS must be formulated and debated in a transparent process that allows PLWHAs and other stakeholders extra opportunity for participation and influence. At the very least, the opportunity for people to choose between alternative political interventions as proposed by contending parties in free and fair elections is paramount.

UNDP 3: People can hold decision-makers accountable.

Idasa 3: Those in power must be answerable for the decisions they take; the citizenry must have the capacity to be able to demand it. A variety of procedural and legal, as well as cultural and social, levers will drive a different relationship between those in power and the governed. We assert that the practice of transparent gov-ernment, backed by effectively implemented "right to know" law and policy, will enable people to demand the highest standards from those in public office. Where decision-makers fail to fulfil promises or implement inefficient policies in the fight against HIV/AIDS, those ultimately responsible must agree to stand down if their (in)actions have undermined their credibility in the eyes of stakeholders or the public in general. A number of institutional arrangements can affect such account-ability, of which free and fair democratic elections is the most common.

UNDP 4: Inclusive and fair rules, institutions and practices govern social interactions.

Idasa 4: The rules of the democratic game must be clear and known; if their origin is inclusive and involves the participation of all major stakeholders in society, they will attain the necessary level of legitimacy to encourage democratic tolerance and respect for the institutions of governance. Key civil and political freedoms, such as the right to freedom of expression and assembly, and the right to administrative justice to counteract abusive or arbitrary use of public power, will create the frame-work for a democratic society. In turn, in the arena of public health, inclusive and fair rules, institutions and practices govern social interactions between those who are and those who are not infected and/or directly affected by HIV and AIDS.

UNDP 5: Women are equal partners with men in private and public spheres of life and deci-sion-making.

Idasa 5: Women have the fundamental right to equality, procedurally and substan-tively. Democracy demands that the rights of women are fully respected and pro-tected. Due to being particularly vulnerable to the epidemic, women's experiences of being directly or indirectly affected by the epidemic must be prioritised in all decision-making.

UNDP 6: People are free from discrimination based on race, ethnicity, class, gender or any other attribute.

Idasa 6: Similarly, the right to equal treatment and protection against unlawful discrimination is fundamental to a modern democracy based on universal norms and standards. The potential stigma of HIV/AIDS raises significant dangers of discrimination. As a means to reduce the stigma attached to HIV/AIDS, the right to non-discrimination for those living with the virus should be elevated to the same level as other fundamental rights given to other categories of the population. HIV/AIDS is of no lesser concern or importance to society as a whole if it mainly affects one or more population segment that is relatively marginalised from power.

UNDP 7: The needs of future generations are reflected in current practices.

Idasa 7: The rights of children that are articulated so clearly in international law must be respected in the national sphere. The principal driver of change in this regard is to ensure that children can enjoy the right to a quality education, and that choices about the allocation of resources prioritises education and takes account of the barriers to the realisation of the right to education, such as food insecurity and inadequate public transportation. By the same token, the different decisions on prioritisation of resources and rights that go into formulating HIV/AIDS policy must also take into consideration the needs of today's AIDS orphans and the sustainability of society beyond their generation.

UNDP 8: Economic and social policies are responsive to people's needs and aspirations.

Idasa 8: The policy-making environment must be geared to permit people and civil society organisations to intervene before policy is finalised. Citizens are the best witnesses to their problems and needs; space must be created to allow their voices to be heard when designing prescriptions. On public health, government policy on HIV/AIDS must adapt in accordance with perceived incidence and estimated prevalence of HIV, and experienced illnesses and deaths from AIDS.

UNDP 9: Economic and social policies aim at eradicating poverty and expanding the choices that all people have in their lives.

Idasa 9: Endemic poverty and chronic unemployment undermine human dignity, drive human insecurity and thereby dilute and threaten the democratic dividend. The eradication of poverty must, therefore, be the number one priority of government, in partnership with all major social stakeholders. On the most vulnerable groups in society, government policy on HIV/AIDS must also address the structural problems that impact on the prevalence of HIV and reduce the receptiveness in people to treatment against AIDS. Only a person who has both information and realistic alternatives is truly empowered to change a behaviour that fuels the epidemic.[58] Given this elaborate background, there are several ways in which the link between HIV/AIDS and democratic governance may be analysed assuming the impact of Anti-Retroviral Therapy (ART) is not optimistically factored-in:

• Growth is stunted through reduced Gross Domestic Product (GDP) as productive citizens die. Household incomes are stretched due to funeral, medical and legal costs. AIDS hence makes a significant contribution to poverty as earning power is lost by the sick and by households with deceased bread winners. The economic security of millions is threatened. Economic under-performance affects citizen confidence in the government of the day and, more critically, in the political system itself. Further, increased AIDS deaths amongst the working class could reduce tax bases and therefore the financial resources available to finance budgets.

- More generally, rising mortality rates may increase demands on public health and welfare expenditure as AIDS continues to infect millions. Health services struggle to cope with this unprecedented load while budgets are stretched beyond limits. Spending on health is highly reliant on donor funding, which raises questions about sustainability and endurance in addressing AIDS as a "long wave" crisis. The health security of nations is compromised.

- Poor economic performance may lead to democratic reversals which happen from time to time: Armed conflict or other forms of destabilisation may lead to economic and social collapse or poor productivity due to loss of skilled labour to more stable economies. Food (security) emergencies may occur and increase vulnerability to HIV as women and men trade sex for scarce commodities. Instances of sexual abuse might also increase the incidence of HIV.

> **Citizens are the best witnesses to their problems and needs.**

- Due to limited availability of antiretroviral drugs, AIDS relief could be apportioned along ethnic or partisan lines, generating tension between working classes and various tribal groups, possibly exacerbating corruption and fomenting dissent amongst the marginalised.

- PLWHAs are targets of violence, including the psychological violence of stigma and discrimination. Gender-based violence increases female vulnerability to HIV infection. People living with AIDS withdraw from the electoral process for fear of violence or due to stigma. Similarly, there is public humiliation of people (perceived) to be living with AIDS who would seek elective office. This phenomenon exacerbates this feeling of personal insecurity.

- With the higher concentration of deaths from AIDS normally in the 15-49 age cohort, there is a strong likelihood that voting age populations will be depleted, affecting participation levels negatively. Millions of potential voters could be constrained by illness and care-giving and could therefore be rendered unable to navigate complex procedural processes that are required for citizen and voter registration. Lack of legitimacy can in turn spawn political conflict and instability as opponents seek legal and illegal means to challenge outcomes.

- AIDS could lead to political opportunism, allowing for leaders with simplistic solutions to manipulate public opinion regardless of whether they uphold democratic governance principles or not.

- The burden of orphans could similarly be overwhelming, not only tearing family systems apart but also stretching the state and civil society's resources. With millions of children in the streets, the possibilities of increased crime could rise.

- Lastly, HIV/AIDS could undermine the effectiveness of democratic institutions due to loss of skills, experienced personnel and reduced productivity. The impact of HIV/AIDS on the political society reduces the capacities of the military, political parties and government departments. Service delivery is affected, resulting in citizen protests. Skilled personnel are depleted from the ranks of electoral management bodies, political parties and parliaments, affecting institutional memory, democratic confidence and integrity. Weak governance increases chances of instability.[59]

We can assume that there will be other related arguments that will galvanise the discourse on governance and AIDS more generally. However our aims in this project are restricted to the institutional capacity and effectiveness of our democratic institutions and the participation of citizens in procedural processes in the face of HIV/AIDS. In the next section, therefore, we begin to illustrate the impact of HIV/AIDS on the central institution of elections and discuss the democratic governance implications that will likely arise as a result of this new knowledge.

Chapter Four: Overview of Findings

The place of the electoral system in governance has been discussed in detail and its sensitivities and democratic relevance articulated at length. We take note that electoral systems come in many forms, can influence different outcomes and may require varying levels of expertise, organisation and financial capacity to sustain. While the criteria for designing electoral models constitute varied elements, in this section we shall focus mainly on the question of sustainability.

1. FPTP, MMP vs PR

Our examination of the First-Past-The-Post (FPTP), Mixed Member Proportional (MMP), Parallel and Proportional Representation (PR) electoral systems indicates clearly that the first two systems, in their current form as instituted in the SADC region, are highly vulnerable to HIV/AIDS.

SADC countries using these two systems have experienced an unusually large proportion of by-elections caused by Members of Parliament (MPs) dying of undisclosed ailments. Because records of the actual causes of deaths of elected representatives are often unavailable, there are a number of steps we have taken to explain the impact of the AIDS pandemic on electoral systems. We have done this by:

- Comparing and analysing trends in the deaths of elected leaders during the "pre-AIDS" period and the "AIDS era";
- Analysing the age cohorts of the deceased leaders (do they fall within the sexually active age group of 20-60 years?);
- And finally aggregating the causes of by-elections in countries that employ the FPTP and MMP systems (was there an increase in the number of by-elections caused by illness in the "AIDS era" compared to the "pre-AIDS era"?).

Although these steps do not conclusively attribute deaths to AIDS they do help us draw inferences on the pattern of deaths and their correlation to trends in AIDS deaths in the national population. High mortality among younger politicians (aged 40-55) provides a strong basis to link the deaths that have been attributed officially to "long" or "short illness" to the influence of the pandemic. Following this we expand the discussion by addressing the political and economic consequences of the pandemic resulting from its effect on the electoral system. These costs are best exemplified by assessing the FPTP and MMP systems which employ by-elections to fill vacancies. It is less useful to use the PR system because vacancies are filled by appointment from the party lists.

1.1 FPTP and MMP countries: Malawi, Tanzania, Zambia and Zimbabwe

We observe that the trends in countries which had severe epidemics in the 1990s, such as Malawi, Tanzania, Zambia and Zimbabwe, reflect a higher level of attrition amongst MPs. We also notice that death far outstrips resignations, defections, retirement or appointments as causes of parliamentary vacancies in countries that are also high-HIV prevalence zones.

We observe that the frequent deaths of MPs and other political representatives as a result of illness have only become commonplace in the last 15 years in Zambia for instance. As a result, the number of by-elections generated by the natural deaths of incumbent MPs and councillors has also increased during the same period. While only 6.44% of the 46 by-elections held between 1964 and 1984 were caused by MPs dying natural deaths, the numbers rose dramatically between 1985 and 2006: in that period at least 60% of the 146 by-elections held were due to deaths of incumbent MPs. It can of course be argued that parliament size changed during that period but that does not discount the fact that the rate of deaths still remains high.

Our research in Malawi also shows that there was a steady rise in the number of legislators who died in the 1994-1996 period – which was the height of the AIDS pandemic – compared to the 1999-2004 period. A total of 42 MPs died between 1994 and 2006. Of the 193 MPs at the end of 2005, 87 (45%) were below 50 years of age and 138 or about 72% were below 60 years of age. These figures suggest that the house is full of people who are still in the prime of their lives and will fall within the "vulnerable" category.

> Zanzibar is a much smaller area to barnstorm with AIDS campaigns.

An official statement in 2000 by the then Speaker of the National Assembly disclosed that 28 MPs in Malawi had died of HIV/AIDS-related complexes. Malawi lost seven MPs in a single year (2005). Twenty three MPs died between 1994 and 1999 and 12 between 1999 and 2004.

In Tanzania, a total of 31 MPs died between 1991 and 2006. As in the other countries, no information is available on the actual cause of death in cases where illness is involved. Four MPs are listed as victims of car accidents and shootings, while the rest died from undisclosed "long" and "short" illnesses. Mortality at the House of Representatives in Zanzibar is relatively low at five deaths between 1990 and 2005. The disparities between Zanzibar (less than 1% prevalence and 4.7 incidence in 2004 (UNAIDS; 2005)), and Tanzania mainland (7% HIV prevalence rate) in terms of prevalence rates might be explained by the influence of religion or geographical position and size, among other things.

Zanzibar is a much smaller area to barnstorm with AIDS campaigns. In addition, deviant behaviour in a place where everybody knows everybody else will very likely be frowned upon. In particular, the influence of Islam coupled with strong management of the pandemic and its link to the spread of HIV/AIDS is a matter requiring further investigation.

There is further evidence provided by Zimbabwe in terms of the instability of the FPTP system in the face of HIV/AIDS. Zimbabwe held its most competitive parlia-

Figure 4.1: Causes of vacancies in national Parliaments

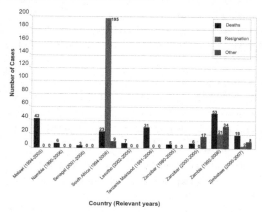

Figure 4.2: Age cohort and numbers of deceased MPs 1990-2003 Zambia

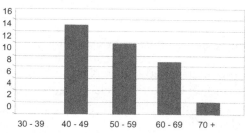

Source: Chirambo, 2003; 2006.

mentary election in 2000, upon the birth of the Movement for Democratic Change (MDC) which rigorously tested the liberation party the Zimbabwe African National Union Patriotic Front (ZANU-PF). The ruling ZANU-PF headed by founding president Robert Mugabe won a relatively slender victory over leader Morgan Tsvangirai's MDC: 62 seats to 57 seats (of 120 elective seats).

A succession of 29 by-elections had been held by 2005, with 19 having been caused by the deaths of MPs as a result of undisclosed illnesses. At least one vacancy was caused by the resignation of an MP on account of ill health, another was appointed to higher office. Additional reasons for the vacancies that led to by-elections were the dismissal of an MP. Six constituencies Buhera North; Hurungwe East; Mutoko South; Chiredzi North; Gokwe North; and Gokwe South had their results nullified by the high court following petitions by losing candidates. The sitting MPs appealed to the Supreme Court but the case was still being heard by the time of the 2005 parliamentary elections.

1.2 THE PARALLEL AND PR SYSTEMS: SENEGAL, NAMIBIA AND SOUTH AFRICA

Senegal generally exhibits prevalence rates among the general population that vary between 0.7% and 9% (UNAIDS, 2006),[60] which is still far below the Sub-Saharan levels. During Senegal's 2001-2006 parliamentary session, only three MPs died. This figure does not indicate a substantial increase in deaths when compared with prior legislatures, particularly those before the HIV/AIDS pandemic. It has also not been established that there has been a high mortality in elected representatives of local government.

In the same vein, Namibia does not show any significant trends that may be linked to an unusual phenomenon such as HIV/AIDS. It may be argued that this is because the Namibia epidemic may be comparatively less severe.[61] Also, data from the apartheid era was not made available to us. Records from the country's parliament indicate that between 1990 and 2006 six sitting MPs died. Four of these were from the National Assembly and two from the National Council. None died from illnesses related to

HIV/AIDS according to the causes of death issued to the media. Press reports at the time of the MPs deaths gave as the causes complications from diabetes, vehicle accident, long and short illnesses and heart attack. The death rates among the 98 elected members of both houses have remained relatively low. As in South Africa, the PR system employed at national level is relatively cheaper to manage when vacancies occur as no by-elections are required.

Data from the parliament of South Africa suggests that 227 MPs departed (resigned, were appointed to higher positions or were dismissed) between 1994 and 2006. Twenty three of the vacancies arose as a result of deaths. There is no information on the causes of deaths and no evidence to suggest that the trends mimic the so-called AIDS mortality profile, where relatively younger people (aged 50 and below) die at a faster rate than relatively older people (50 and over). The relatively lower death rates have been explained as to do with the extent of medical cover extended to parliamentarians in South Africa.[62]

While this might be a factor, it should also be noted that other countries also have similar medical aid schemes. But the fact that senior parliamentarians from other SADC states have on occasion been flown to South Africa or abroad for advanced medical attention in some instances indicates a disparity in the capacity and quality of medical care.[63]

1.3 MMP: LESOTHO AND SOUTH AFRICA (LOCAL GOVERNMENT)

While South Africa appears insulated from the financial costs of replacing deceased leaders, it has held by-elections at a local level to replace directly elected councillors under the MMP system employed at the local government level. The electoral system used for local government elections is as follows: (a) for local and municipal councils (Category A and Category B respectively) 50% of ward councillors are elected directly through the FPTP system and the other 50% through the PR model in order to achieve overall political proportionality; and (b) at the district level (Category C) 40% of the councillors are directly elected by eligible district residents while 60% of the councillors are indirectly elected in that they are appointed representatives of local and municipal councils (Strand, Strode, Matlosa & Chirambo: 2005).

In 2001, a total of 79 by-elections were held. Of these 27 were in KwaZulu-Natal and nine in Gauteng. A study undertaken by Michael Sachs[64] provides reasons for the by-elections held by province. The Sachs report indicates that of the 79 by-elections in 2001, 34 were caused by a councillor's resignation, 33 resulted from the death of a councillor and 12 were the result of the expulsion of a councillor either from the party or the council concerned. It has to be stated that in Africa, generally, MPs and councillors will enjoy a much higher standard of living than the general population and will also have access to better medical services. These deaths would have occurred despite all that.

To further underline the vulnerability of the MMP system we turn to the Kingdom of Lesotho where deaths amongst MPs and other factors continue to generate costly by-elections despite a change in the electoral model. Eight by-elections were held in the kingdom between 2002 and 2005, the period in which the modified MMP electoral model was instituted.[65] Seven of the MPs had been elected through the FPTP system and one through the PR system.

2. AVERAGE AGES OF MPS AND VULNERABILITY FACTORS

Nuances in this discussion suggest that the younger MPs are the more vulnerable and will continue to be susceptible in the absence of holistic strategies to maintain a relatively AIDS-free future leadership. On the basis of the current information provided by the respective national assemblies, Zambia has the youngest parliamentarians on average at 46 years; followed by Namibia and Malawi at 51 years, Tanzania has a relatively higher average of 54, while South Africa and Senegal come in at 55 years.

In analysing the ages of the parliamentarians in relation to their vulnerability to HIV/AIDS, we need to bear in mind that the epidemic is "a long wave event". We started discussing its trajectory from the mid-1980s when most countries recorded their first cases. This was a time when HIV risk perception would have been relatively low in the general population and the leadership. This phase was followed by long periods of denial by many countries around the globe as to the extent of the epidemic amongst their people. Stigma and discrimination were rife; ignorance and myths predominant.

> It is highly likely that many of the older MPs who may have died of AIDS in the 1990s contracted the virus in the early 1980s.

This would have been the phase in which most of the parliamentarians who were 40 years old in 1987 for instance will be 60 years old today. In short, it may be naïve of us to simply categorise 18-49-year-olds in the present day as being potential casualties of HIV/AIDS. It is highly likely that many of the older MPs who may have died of AIDS in the 1990s contracted the virus in the early 1980s. Therefore, a person who is in their sixties by 1999 or in the next millennium might quite easily have carried the virus leading to their eventual death.

In Zambia for instance, we see a concentration of deaths amongst the 40-49 and 50-59 age cohort between 1990 and 2003. Most of these people would have been younger and vibrant in the 1980s and therefore more vulnerable to HIV/AIDS given their presumably more sexually active lifestyles at the time. This was the period in which ARV access was almost non-existent. In the rare situations when it was available much later in the late 1990s, it was prohibitively expensive.

To underline this point, we turn to the experience of one of the champions of HIV/AIDS in the world today. Judge Edwin Cameron of South Africa is the only high-profile figure to disclose his HIV status. Unlike the subjects of this study, he is not an elected official. He was born on 15 February, 1953.[66] He disclosed his status in 1999 when he was 46 years old during a job interview with the Judicial Service Commission. A high court judge at the Supreme Court of Appeal, Cameron was 54 in 2007 and by his own assertion, has had the benefit of treatment, job security and support of family, friends and colleagues, factors that could explain his longevity as a PLWHA.[67] There would have been many less fortunate citizens and political elites within the SADC region who had limited or no access to ARVs, particularly in the early to mid-1990s.

3   LOSS OF REPRESENTATION

The immediate political cost of the death of an MP is the constituency's loss of representation. Depending on the time it takes to replace the deceased through by-elections, this might disadvantage the masses. MPs are expected to drive development at constituency level, even though they may not always have the resources to do so. Any long period without representation alienates the affected districts. On the Tanzania mainland, six constituencies Kisesa, Mbeya Vijijini, Ulanga Mashariki, Kasulu Mashariki, Rahaleo and Kilombero had no MPs by the December 2005 general elections. Their MPs had died during the 2000-2005 parliamentary sitting. During the 1995-2000 parliaments, ten MPs died.

In Malawi, it took more than a year for by-elections to be conducted in the six constituencies that fell vacant after the 2004 elections. Lack of finances is understood to be the main reason. The lack of capacity of Malawi to finance elections from its own vault was revealed when local government elections scheduled for 2005 were postponed. A crunching food security crisis for the predominantly agrarian economy meant that the state was unable to raise enough funds to support its local polls, resulting in a constitutional crisis. In the case of parliamentary vacancies, the requirement by law is that a by-election be held within 90 days of a seat being declared vacant. The MEC is required to prepare special budgets to justify central treasury funding, which are often not approved in time. Hence, the reality is that the timeframes for holding by-elections have not been adhered to. The implication of this is that the voices of ordinary people, often expressed through vibrant elected representatives, are silenced for an unusually long time. In cases where an MP is also responsible for assisting in donor and state interventions in community-based projects, the benefit to the constituency may be affected by his/her absence.

A very real consideration of the prospect of too many by-elections within months or weeks of each other is poor attendance by the electorate. Voting consumes a substantial amount of an individual's time; it can be frustrating to spend long periods in queues or at a campaign rally. Poor turnouts will raise problems of legitimacy for the winners as they may be seen to represent only relatively few people.

4   PARLIAMENTS: CHANGING POWER CONFIGURATIONS IN NATIONAL PARLIAMENTS OF ZAMBIA AND ZIMBABWE

We note that disease in general, and HIV/AIDS in particular, contributes to power shifts in countries operating the FPTP electoral model. This phenomenon is best exemplified by Zambia and Zimbabwe where elections have become increasingly competitive. The effect of natural deaths, combined with vacancies generated by expulsions, resignations or floor-crossing by members, compelled Zimbabwe to hold 14 by-elections following the 2000 legislative polls. Eight of the by-elections arose because parliamentary representatives had died prematurely of undisclosed illnesses.

In the 2000 Zimbabwean parliamentary elections ZANU-PF won 62 seats of the 120 elective seats while the opposition MDC secured 57 seats. A lone seat went to the other opposition ZANU-Ndonga party. Through victories in most by-elections, ZANU-PF increased its parliamentary strength from 62 to 67 seats by 2004. It secured five extra seats from the MDC whose portfolio shrank within the same period from 57 to 52 seats.

Figure 4.3 Seats breakdown per Parliament

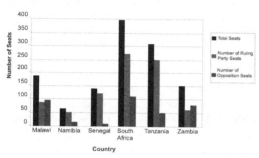

Source: Malawi, Namibia, Senegal, South Africa, Tanzania and Zambia parliaments. Compiled by Idasa.

Death has now become the biggest cause of vacancies in the Zimbabwe parliament. Between 2004 and 2007, 19 of the 29 by-elections held were due to MPs dying from undisclosed illnesses. The effect of numerous by-elections is that the opposition parties have generally lost the majority of the polls, partly perhaps due to their inability to compete with a well-resourced ruling party. In Zambia, the opposition also lost ground after entering parliament in the 2001 general elections with a combined slender majority. The by-elections that followed in succession several months later were won mainly by the ruling Movement for Multi-party Democracy (MMD). There is nothing undemocratic about this, one might add. But it is an important observation regarding how a disease may contribute to tipping the balance of power.

For example, table 4.1 indicates that of the 29 by-elections held between 26 June 2001 and 12 April 2006, the ruling MMD gained 14 seats from the opposition out of a pool of 16 held by the opposition following the general elections of 2001.

Thus the MMD's strength increased from 46% to 54% representation in parliament between the 2001 and the 2006 presidential and parliamentary general elections.

Table 4.1: Power shifts in Zambian parliament between 2001 and 2006									
	MMD	UPND	FDD	UNIP	HP	PF	ZRP	INDPT	Totals
2001 election seats	69 (46%)	49 (32.7%)	12 (8%)	13 (8.7%)	4 (2.7%)	1 (0.7%)	1 (0.7%)	1 (0.7%)	150 (100%)
Seats lost	2	7	1	4	2	1	0	0	15
Seats retained	11	1	0	0	0	1	0	0	13
Seats gained	14	0	1	0	0	1	0	0	16
Net gain	12	-6	0	-4	-2	0	0	0	
Pre-2006 election seats	81 (54%)	43 (28.7%)	12 (8%)	9 (6%)	2 (1.3%)	1 (0.7%)	1 (0.7%)	1 (0.7%)	150 (100%)
Source: Foundation for Democratic Process									

Conversely, the parliamentary representation of the two larger opposition parties that could present the stiffest challenge to the MMD in general elections, the UPND and UNIP, dropped from 49% to 43% and 8.7% to 6% respectively. These two examples clearly show how numerous by-elections, whether generated by HIV/AIDS or not, are likely to favour the ruling parties and significantly alter the balance of power. This, as asserted above, would impact on political party policy leverage determining governance priorities.

5. ECONOMIC COSTS

There is a high cost to the Treasury in holding numerous by-elections. In December 2005 the six by-elections in Malawi cost an estimated MK65 million ($US474 799.12), which translated into approximately MK10.8 million ($US78 889.70) per constituency. Each by-election held in Zambia cost US$235,849 on average.[68] In Tanzania, by-elections cost between $US300 000 and $US500 000 depending on the size of the voting district. The MMP in Lesotho is equally vulnerable: the seven by-elections held in Lesotho since the country modified the electoral model in 2002 from FPTP to an MMP system each cost approximately R1million (US$143 601[69]). Three by-elections were the result of the deaths of MPs. Although wards are smaller and therefore less costly, the cumulative effect of holding many by-elections in terms of South Africa's MMP system at local government level could prove daunting. A ward poll can cost approximately R30 000.00 ($4000 at the rand-US dollar exchange rate at the time of writing).[70] Countries such as Malawi and Zambia have had their national elections substantially supported in financial terms by foreign donors, which may render the prospect of increased by-elections more onerous.[71]

Table 4.2: Average cost of by-elections		
Country	Electoral system	Average cost of by-elections
Tanzania mainland	FPTP	US$416.000
Zanzibar	FPTP	US$45,000
Zambia	FPTP	US$235,849
Malawi	FPTP	US$78,889
Lesotho	MMP	US$143,601[72]
Source: Compiled by Idasa		

The costs illustrated above only relate to the state's allocations to the EMB. These costs will cover the provision of air/road transport to deliver ballots; design and printing of ballots; setting up temporary shelters for electoral staff; allowances for election and presiding officers; lighting for the polling stations; booths; communication; advertising on television, radio and newspapers; posters; public education of a direct nature; discursive programmes for political parties, among other things.

Table 4.2 does not include costs incurred by civil society and donor agencies for election monitoring and voter and civic education activities. Nor does it include expenditure by political parties on repeated campaigns. Finances will be needed by parties to cover road/air transport; television and newspaper advertising; public meetings; salaries or stipends for support staff and cadres; t-shirts for promoting candidates; paying political party monitors, among other things. Cash-strapped political parties will obviously be outpaced by the more powerful entities. If neither the competing political parties or the civil society monitors are able to achieve sufficient coverage of all electoral events, the likelihood of post-election conflict might rise as independent voices and "judges" will be seen to be absent from the electoral process, undermining the credibility of the outcomes.

6. PARLIAMENTARY DEBATES ON HIV/AIDS

Despite the now rather distinct manner in which elected MPs have been dying in countries severely affected by AIDS, we do not see any significant levels of debate within parliament that suggests that the institutions have even attempted to investigate mortality amongst their members let alone deploy in-house strategies to minimise the impact. Parliaments in Namibia, Malawi, Tanzania, Senegal, South Africa and Zambia have interrogated many aspects of the HIV pandemic, including high costs, drugs, rape and deliberate transmission of the HI virus, orphaning, behaviour change, preventative methods, budget allocations and culture, among other things. While evidence exists that MPs in Tanzania for instance have encouraged each other to go for VCT, there is no public disclosure or records of how many have actually volunteered for tests.

The high attrition rates from death within parliaments has not however been lost on some publics: the Medical Association of Zambia initiated a debate on mandatory HIV testing for all presidential and parliamentary candidates in 2005, as the country's 2006 general elections approached. Despite the media storm that followed, relatively lukewarm responses in terms of parliamentary discussions were observed. Human rights activists argued that such a move would violate the rights of MPs.

And while Senegalese MPs interviewed for this study profess to be actively involved in HIV/AIDS initiatives in their local communities, the parliament does not have institutionalised approaches to deal with members who are PLWHAs. The low prevalence status of Senegal might encourage a sense of low risk perception as exemplified by the MP who remarked that AIDS does not constitute a major priority: "At this moment, it must all the same be recognised that sectors like education, agriculture and the fight against poverty have priority over the other ones..."

The debate on VCT for elected representatives also emerged in Namibia. Former

Figure 4.4: Average cost of national elections per voter

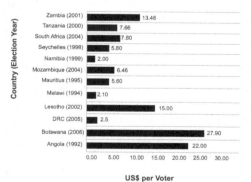

Source: EISA 2006; Idasa: 2002

Swapo MP, Ben Ulenga, who was Deputy Minister of Local Government at the time, stirred a heated debate when he announced his intention in 1996 to take a test for HIV. He also alleged that half the national parliament was infected by the virus. His negative results did not inspire others to follow suit. In the seven countries being studied that have released preliminary results, there is not a single elected member or cabinet minister known to be HIV-positive. This contradicts the statistics just presented.

The South African parliament is also cagey on the matter. Perhaps what is even more surprising is that Malawi, a country whose speaker was on record as having attributed 28 of the 31 deaths amongst MPs (by the year 2000) to AIDS-related illness, does not appear to have had any significant reference to the impact of the epidemic on the national assembly and its representatives. Such blatant disregard may quite easily be interpreted as denial. This denial may be a direct result of stigma and discrimination in politics otherwise referred to herein as "political stigma".

6.1 POLITICAL OSTRACISM AND POLITICAL RIGHTS

In all the countries studied, there appears to be an inherent fear of disclosure due to the potential loss of economic benefits that come with being a politician. Disclosure of one's HIV status has been equated with "political suicide" or becoming "a political liability" to the party. A salient feature noted in our research in Zambia is the use of HIV/AIDS as a weapon in electoral politics. Opposition candidates who are perceived to be sick are undermined and destroyed before the eyes of the electorate. Weight loss is closely associated with AIDS and has caused opposition parties to cast doubt on the health of leading candidates and incumbents alike. In our post-research stakeholder meetings with the ruling MMD and opposition parties in July 2006 in Zambia this was further underlined by top party officials. No party was willing to adopt a candidate who was HIV-positive or was perceived to be positive, as they were seen to be liabilities (Chirambo: 2006). In Malawi, some political party candidates were reluctant to dwell on HIV/AIDS during the campaign for the 2004 presidential and parliamentary elections for fear of being associated with the illness. Senegalese MPs were equally reluctant to pursue an open policy on their HIV status. As indicated in the foregoing, Namibia and Tanzania are not any different.

> Disclosure of one's HIV status has been equated with "political suicide".

We take note therefore of the silent exclusionary practices of political elites who have taken to marginalising fellow aspirants to elective office at the remotest sign of illness. Political ostracism should, in our view, be considered a real threat to people's political rights. It has led to the highly improbable record of non-disclosure amongst senior elected officials in government and parliamentary structures. To date, no elected official is on record as carrying HIV, presumably for fear of rejection by their political parties and the electorate. Particularly, pervasive denialism amongst leaders severely undermines their moral authority to address HIV/AIDS as a public policy emergency.[73]

Generally, pervasive denialism permeates societies at all levels. These are matters that require the help of high-level actors to generate a new wave of sensitisation in the echelons of power and start regional and national attitude shifts amongst elites.

7. IMPACT OF HIV/AIDS ON ELECTORAL MANAGEMENT, ADMINISTRATION IN AFRICA

The impact of HIV/AIDS on EMBs has to be understood in three ways:
- The loss of core staff, which might affect efficiency and institutional memory;
- The loss of part-time staff who were mainly drawn from the public service's teaching profession compromises continuity, undermines the quality of work and raises costs as training is then needed for new staff;
- The rapid rise in numbers of deaths renders the voters' roll unmanageable.

Studies are showing a severe impact of AIDS on the public sector and in particular the teaching profession. An estimated 200 000 of Sub-Saharan Africa's 650 000 teachers are projected to die of AIDS. At least half of the positions in the education sector are vacant at present. It is suggested that globally it will cost up to $1billion annually to compensate for the loss and absenteeism of teachers resulting from AIDS.

The sum effect of AIDS on the teaching profession is summarised as follows:
- Infected teachers lose six months of professional working time before developing full-blown AIDS;
- Teachers experience on average 18 months of increasing disability prior to leaving the school system.

The wholesale loss of teachers has wider implications for the affected countries. Firstly, experts assert that the teaching profession constitutes the largest segment of public workers, the public sector being the largest employer in Africa. The attrition of teachers, including university professors, means the next generation of young people will be exposed to poorer quality education. Younger citizens will also find it exceedingly difficult to meet the requirements of highly competitive job markets or will experience difficulties in launching their own entrepreneurships.[74]

In Zambia, it is projected that the HIV/AIDS epidemic is likely to reduce the number of teachers from an expected 59 500 to only 50 000 by 2010, while teacher absenteeism due to HIV-related illnesses will cost 12 450 teacher/years over the next decade. Studies by the Human Sciences Research Council (HSRC) in South Africa indicate that 4 000 teachers died in 2004 while 45 000 more, about 12.7% of the workforce, were HIV-positive. Of those who died of AIDS, 80% were under the age of 45. The study was conducted at 1 700 schools. Ten thousand of the 45 000 HIV-positive teachers needed ARVs (The Star, 05/04/05). A study titled "The Impact of HIV/AIDS on the Human Resources in Malawi's Public Sector" conducted by the Malawi Institute of Management (MIM) for the government of Malawi and the UNDP illustrates a grave situation of morbidity, absenteeism and attrition due to HIV/AIDS among civil servants.

Except for Namibia, where the Electoral Management Body (EMB) advertises temporary work to the general public to assist in elections, the other SADC countries in this study usually utilise teachers for backup during the polls. As conducting elections requires experienced staff, the vulnerability of support personnel to the disease is likely to reduce the Independent Electoral Committee's ability to rely on them to bring their accumulated experience and skills to bear on future elections.

8. IMPACT OF HIV/AIDS ON VOTER REGISTERS

8 1 INSTITUTIONALISED CITIZEN AND VOTER REGISTRATION SYSTEMS

"The impact of HIV/AIDS has forced electoral management bodies to face a number of problems regarding the voters' roll. The number of registered voters on the voters' roll is not a true reflection of what is on the ground. Our voters' rolls are bloated with dead voters." M. Ngwembe, Commissioner Malawi Electoral Commission (Chirambo & Caesar, 2003. p. 128).[75]

The countries in this study have varying levels of development in terms of their electoral institutions. Some, like Tanzania, only established a voters' roll in 2005. Others, like Malawi, have highly controversial rolls that cannot be reconciled with the country's population size, particularly with their Voting Age Population (VAP). Zambia has changed registers at least three times in two decades and only launched a biometric system in 2006. For a long time, the Zambian citizen registration and voter registration systems have not been directly compatible; they are two different processes that are independently managed. Senegal also instituted a digitised citizen ID and voter registration mechanism in 2007. South Africa has a technologically advanced and well established citizen and voter registration systems which allows it to timeously remove dead voters from the registers. Rather than compare systems that are in effect incomparable, we choose to contrast the problems associated with not having an institutionalised citizen and voter registration system in the age of AIDS with the benefits of investing in one. In this regard, we contrast Malawi with South Africa.

MALAWI

The case of Malawi is a compelling one in as far as defining how a country struggling with the installation of a credible citizen, voter and death registration system is challenged to deal with high attrition rates amongst its population. Firstly, the death registration system in Malawi is at best colonial. When citizens in rural outposts die, their deaths are relayed to the chiefs and it is through them that confirmation of death is captured by the government. This system will not respond expeditiously to the high attrition associated with AIDS. This will lead to the electoral roll, which should eliminate the names of all registered voters on receipt of a death certificate, to be highly unreliable. In the 1999 general elections, the Malawi Electoral Commission registered 5 071 822 voters. The MEC claimed to have removed 106 086 registered voters from the roll in the five years prior to the 2004 general elections. A highly disputed figure of 6 668 839 registered voters was announced for 18 May 2004 presidential and parliamentary elections, despite the removal of dead voters.[76]

The National Statistics Office (NSO) projections during the same period suggested that there were 5 594 081 people aged 18 years or older in Malawi who were eligible to vote. In short, the MEC could not adequately explain where the extra one million registered voters came from.

> "Our projections [based on the last (1998/99) national population census] are [that] the population has grown at an average rate of 3.2 per cent", observed the NSO. [sic:] "But if you calculate the average rates at which the Commission's figures are based, you will find that they are way above the normal population growth rate."

Mainly because of the system's failure to account for all its citizens and its voters, dead or alive, the results of Malawi's 2004 elections were highly controversial especially as the eventual president, Dr Bingu Wa Mutharika, won by a slender majority with an opposition-controlled parliament. The results have led to the relatively weak mandate that Mutharika has had to endure, surviving several impeachment initiatives by the opposition in the process.

SOUTH AFRICA

The case of South Africa is radically different. Equipped with bar-coded IDs and with electronic compatibility between citizen and voter registers, South Africa purges dead voters on a monthly basis. The dataset from the Independent Electoral Commission in South Africa contains the following:

The number of registered voters at the end of 1999, 2000, 2001, 2002 and 2003; the total number of deceased registered voters for 1999, 2000, 2001, 2002 and 2003, for each gender and each age cohort (18–19; 20–29; 30–39: 40–49; 50–59; 60–69; 70–79; 80+); the number of registered voters at the end of 1999, 2000, 2001, 2002 and 2003, for each gender, each age cohort (as above), each province and each municipality; and the total number of deceased registered voters for 1999, 2000, 2001, 2002 and 2003, for each gender, each age cohort (as above), each province and each municipality.

The data is extremely powerful as it provides absolute numbers of deceased voters at all levels of governance. Based on this dataset, it was established in our South African study that 1 488 242 of the country's registered voters died between 1999 and 2003 out of a total of 20 674 926 people who were on the voters' roll for the 2004 general elections. Deaths are concentrated in the 20-49 years and 60-79 years age groups. We argue that the sharp increases in mortality in some cases up to

Figure 4.5: South Africa: Increase (in %) in relative numbers of deaths among registered voters 1999-2003, per age and sex

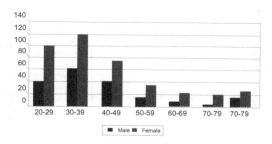

Source: IEC

Matrix of electoral management systems in SADC and Senegal

	Malawi	Namibia	Senegal	South Africa	Tanzania	Zambia
Citizen registration system	No citizen register Death registration not institutionalised (done by local chief).	National identity card.	New digitised ID system introduced.	Digitised bar coded ID system.	National ID system available.	ID system available.
Voter registration system	Voter register available but size unknown (controversial).	Voter register available.	New biometric register established in 2006.	Digitised electoral register.	No register until 2005 when Permanent Voters Register was introduced.	New biometric register introduced in 2006.
Purging of dead voters	Problematic and slow because the country does not have a civic register. However, each voter's status must be verified by a district commissioner, village headman, chief or other prominent person.	It is provided that monthly updates should be made but this has shown to be ineffective and not constant, especially in rural areas.	Until 2000, there was continuous registration. This process did not fully account for deceased voters or changes to voters' personal details. For the 2007 election, the Interior Ministry made a new register. Each Senegalese citizen who meets the legal requirements has to obtain a voter's card and national identity card.	The Independent Electoral Commission (IEC) of South Africa assures us that all dead voters were purged from the voters' roll before the 2004 elections.	Deaths are reported to village chiefs and to home affairs ministry.	The ECZ removes illegally registered persons, dead people or those who change locations. In this system, any citizen or relative can go to the ECZ to lodge a request to remove an individual from the voters' roll citing reasons, including death or ineligibility as in the case of foreigners.
Delimitation of constituencies	The Malawi Electoral Commission is responsible for the demarcation of constituency boundaries and this is contained in Section 72(2) of the Constitution and the Electoral Commission act of 1998 S. 8 (1) Article 106 on Regional Council Elections states that: (1) Each region shall be divided into constituencies ... provided that there shall be no fewer than six and no more than twelve constituencies in each region.	Article 106 on Regional Council Elections states that (1) Each region shall be divided into constituencies the boundaries of which shall be fixed by the Delimitation Commission in accordance with the provisions of an Act of Parliament and this Constitution: provided that there shall be no fewer than six and no more than 12 constituencies in each region.	According to the law, the CENA sets up departments, the embassies and the consulates reporting structures in the regions that can help them fulfil their mandate. In the past (for the 2000 elections), the ONEL had created 10 regional bodies and 40 departmental ones on top of which they themselves nominated 9 000 delegates to represent them in each polling station.	The Electoral Commission Act 51 of 1996 states in chapter 2 (5) (1)(m) that the IEC's functions include the demarcation of wards in the local sphere of government or to cause them to be demarcated.	Article 75(1) (3) and (4) of the Constitution of the United Republic of Tanzania empowers the NEC to demarcate the URT into constituencies and to review the delimitation of constituencies at least once every 10 years.	In terms of Article 77 [Constituencies and Elections]: (1) Zambia shall be divided into constituencies, for purposes of elections to the National Assembly so that the number of such constituencies, the boundaries of which shall be such as an Electoral Commission prescribes, shall be equal to the number of seats of elected members in the Assembly.

	Malawi	Namibia	Senegal	South Africa	Tanzania	Zambia
Establishment of electoral commission	The Constitution of Malawi mandates the establishment of an Electoral Commission that is independent of any external authority (Constitution 1994, Articles 75, 76(4)). The Electoral Commission Act 1998 provides for the setting up of the Malawi Electoral Commission (MEC)	Through the promulgation of the Electoral Act (Act No. 24 of 1992) the ECN was established to direct, supervise and control national, regional and local elections in a fair and impartial manner.	In 2005, a law establishing the Autonomous National Electoral Commission (CENA) was passed. The CENA is a permanent structure with legal status including some financial autonomy. It is responsible for enforcing the electoral law to ensure the transparency of the vote by guaranteeing the free expression of the rights of both voters and candidates.	The IEC was established as an interim body with the mandate to organise and rule on the "freeness and fairness" of the 1994 elections. It was then made a permanent body through the Electoral Commission Act, No. 51 of 1996 to strengthen, promote and safeguard constitutional democracy through the delivery of free and fair elections where voters are able to record their informed choices.	The National Electoral Commission (NEC) is an autonomous government institution. It was established in 1993 under Article 74(1) of the Constitution of the United Republic of Tanzania, 1977.	In terms of Article 76 [Electoral Commission]: (1) The President shall ... establish an Electoral Commission to supervise the registration of voters and the conduct of the Presidential and Parliamentary elections and to review the boundaries of the constituencies into which Zambia is divided for the purposes of elections to the National Assembly.
Appointment of electoral commission officials	The Commission is chaired by a judge nominated by the Judicial Service Commission but appointed by the State President. There are six other commissioners nominated by political parties but appointed by the State President for a four-year renewable term.	The ECN is headed by five commissioners who have been appointed by the President.	The CENA is managed by a President assisted by a vice president and general secretary and includes twelve members. Its members are selected from independent authorities known for their moral integrity, their intellectual honesty and their impartiality.	Five commissioners who have been appointed in terms of par. 6 of the Electoral Act. (Electoral Commission Act, No. 51 of 1996).	The Commission has seven members appointed by the President. The Chairman of the Commission must be either a judge of the High Court or of the Court of Appeal.	The Commission consists of a Chairperson and not more than four other members appointed by the President, subject to ratification by the National Assembly (Section 4 (1) (b)), for a term not exceeding seven years.
Recruitment of temporary staff of electoral commission	The Commission does not have a permanent structure. At elections, Returning Officers are appointed and in most cases District Commissioners act as Returning Officers. To conduct elections efficiently, the MEC relies on the large pool of public servants.	To conduct elections, the ECN appoints Returning Officers, Counting Officers and Presiding Officers. During elections members of the team supporting the election management body are recruited mainly among teachers and public executives.	The members of the team of support to the body of management of elections are recruited mainly among teachers and middle public executives.	In terms of recruiting temporary staff to assist with elections the IEC has a formal arrangement with the Department of Education so that 98% of the presiding officers and deputy presiding officers are drawn from the ranks of teachers.	There are 58 permanent staff members of the NEC. However, during election time the number grows to around 90; some people are taken from other government departments to do temporary work for the Commission.	The ECZ usually hires a temporary workforce from the Local Authorities, the Ministry of Education and other government ministries and departments countrywide to carry out electoral functions as and when the need arises.
Voting age	18	18	18	18	18	18
Source: Country reports; compiled by Idasa						

200% among registered voters between the ages of 20-49, particularly among women in the 30-39 year bracket, can to a large extent, if not wholly, be explained by AIDS.

We based our argument on the strong correspondence between the profiles that our analysis generated and those that have been described by the expert demographers in the field of HIV/AIDS.

NAMIBIA AND SENEGAL

In Namibia, while no evidence of voter attrition to the extent exhibited by South Africa exists, there are strong perceptions by political actors, particularly the opposition, that AIDS has had some influence on the electoral process but there is no empirical evidence to support this belief. The Congress of Democrats (CoD) was concerned that the voters' roll would be outdated due to the high death rates caused by HIV/AIDS. The CoD insists that the Electoral Commission of Namibia (ECN) undertake "immediate and consistent" updating of the roll, rather than "waiting to the last minute" before an election.[77] Delays in dealing with dead electors will escalate if left unattended, the CoD argues. Both the UDF and CoD are in agreement that HIV/AIDS was negatively affecting voter turnout, pointing to bedridden, hospital-bound potential voters who would be marginalised, for instance. In Senegal, the scenario is less compelling as based on the estimated prevalence rate of 1% among adults the number of PLWHAs on voter registers would be insignificant.

9. IMPACT OF HIV/AIDS ON POLITICAL PARTIES

9.1 IMPLICATIONS FOR PARTY STRUCTURES

We stated earlier that there were three levels at which HIV/AIDS may impact on political party structures:

- Organisational: The loss of cadres and members affects electioneering capacity;
- Financial: Loss of members reduces subscriptions;
- Leadership: The loss of a patron can spell the end of a party or compromise its electoral viability and financial status.

The single common feature emerging from preliminary research on political parties in several of the six countries studied is poor record-keeping amongst the entities. Membership cards are often distributed without charge; therefore using a decline in subscription as a proxy indicator for member attrition is futile. However perceptions of loss to HIV/AIDS amongst members are expressed in Namibia, Malawi, Zambia and South Africa by party and government officials alike.

> It is now an acknowledged fact that political parties, which are an essential part of any multi-party democracy, are affected by HIV/AIDS. Almost all political parties in this country have been losing leaders at various levels due to HIV/AIDS-related illness and deaths.[78]

In our 2005 study, the leading political parties in South Africa, including the African

National Congress (ANC), the Democratic Alliance (DA) and the Inkatha Freedom Party (IFP), did acknowledge that HIV/AIDS does or could strain party structures, creating an increased need to replace cadres who have died, especially HIV/AIDS. Although no discernible functional defects have arisen in the party structures, a loss of seniority and experience was reported. A more direct impact acknowledged by religious-based parties such as the African Christian Democratic Party (ACDP) is the time HIV/AIDS-related deaths have committed political leaders to in terms of officiating at recurrent funerals of cadres. This might affect their organisational capacities.

Malawi provides some data on attrition in the structures of its founding party, the Malawi Congress Party (MCP). Confidential correspondence shows that the party lost at least 22 members of its district committees, at least 13 members of its regional committees and not fewer than eight members of its central executive committee between 1987 and 1993. In Senegal, an analysis of parties' programmes and structures shows a poor interest in matters relating to AIDS and health (political parties lack specific structures relating to health and HIV/AIDS issues). During the 2007 presidential campaign, only one candidate mentioned AIDS in a public declaration. This is explained by the low prevalence of HIV in the West African country.

In Namibia nearly all the party spokespeople interviewed indicated that HIV/AIDS has affected their campaign capacity with the loss of key activists, organisers or candidates. The Democratic Turnhalle Alliance's (DTA's) Secretary-General Gende[79] acknowledged that the party's administration had been "dysfunctional", because "highly skilled officials who had been trained through NGOs and the party throughout the years had passed away or were sick in bed and cannot perform." The United Democratic Front (UDF)'s Goreseb[80] underlined that "even the death of one party activist is a notable loss" and could stretch the limited resources of small political parties. Some of the strongholds of the South West African People's Organisation (Swapo), the ruling party, will have been depleted of potential supporters. Areas such as the Caprivi Strip have the highest prevalence rates at 42.6% and are also predominantly controlled by Swapo in terms of voting proclivities.

In Tanzania, political parties foresee the epidemic as having a much larger impact on them in the future and since they do not have the mechanisms to track its impact within party structures, they believe it is a problem requiring strategic planning and further research.

10. IMPACT OF HIV/AIDS ON POLITICAL PARTICIPATION

10.1 STIGMA, DISCRIMINATION AS IMPEDIMENTS TO CITIZEN PARTICIPATION

Finally we come to the "side effects" of AIDS in our societies: stigma and discrimination. Stigmatisation is defined by UNAIDS as "a process of devaluation within a particular culture or setting where attitudes are seized upon and defined as discreditable or not worthy" (Panos/Unicef, 2004). Essentially this means a group of people are cast aside based on the assumption that they are different or apart from the normal social order. It connotes a sense of shame arising from the apparent violation of a set of values or norms by an individual or group. Discrimination is the exclusion that follows this process and can be institutional in character.

AIDS sickness has been highlighted in Tanzania, Zambia, Namibia, Malawi and South Africa as an impediment to political participation. Although the levels of stigma and discrimination differ from country to country, it was only in South Africa that PLWHAs expressed fears about their status compromising their engagement with the wider public in an election. We can explain this by appreciating the mature nature of the epidemic in other African countries, where longer periods of living with the epidemic may have led to greater awareness within their communities. Also, the higher literacy levels would explain higher levels of tolerance.

In our South Africa study, stigma and discrimination resonated as the single most dominant determinants of lack of participation in elections by PLWHAs and care-givers in rural KwaZulu-Natal. Focus group discussions with PLWHAs and caregivers, who were all registered voters for the 2004 election in urban and rural areas of KwaZulu-Natal, yielded seemingly well-founded fears that communities will further ostracise or marginalise those infected and affected if they appeared at major public events. The participants' opinions are corroborated by the findings of studies on stigma and discrimination, particularly the South African Department of Health study of 2002, that HIV/AIDS remains a taboo topic among some South African communities, especially in the rural enclaves. The sense of stigma, it seems, is strongest where people are symptomatic; participants said that most members of the communities would not stand in the same queue with someone with visible signs of disease e.g. body rashes or sores. Although we cannot say how many people stayed away due to AIDS, the disparities between turnout and Voting Age Population present further opportunities for us to interrogate the gaps in registration and voting and the underlying causes.

> Assessments of voter turnouts can be misleading because they are calculated against registered voters.

Quite often, as stated earlier, assessments of voter turnouts are misleading because they are calculated against registered voters. In such instances, even when registration levels are low, the turnout may appear high. However, when turnout is calculated as a percentage of Voting Age Population, we get a much more comprehensive picture of participation. The figures below clearly show these disparities.

Based on these discussions, we concluded that in South Africa people who have visible signs of HIV/AIDS and those who have publicly declared their status are more likely to withdraw from public voting, particularly if they are located in a rural area. There is nothing to suggest that PLWHAs have lost the will to participate in political life. In fact, the majority of participants expressed a desire to participate but said they were constrained by attitudinal and structural factors. Structural factors included lack of transport, toilets, seating facilities and running water at polling stations. These results are not representative of the opinions of all PLWHAs but they are indicative of such attitudes across several countries. It needs to be reiterated that the value of qualitative studies is in the depth and wealth of information that is drawn from our units of analysis rather than the number of people involved in the discussions or interviews.

10.2 PUBLIC OPINION

The Afrobarometer network, in its Compendium of Trends in Public Opinion in 12 African countries, provides useful insights into citizen perceptions of government performance on meeting key governance indicators including health and HIV/AIDS. The barometer conducted its round one surveys between July 1999 and March 2001; round two surveys between May 2002 and September 2003; and round three surveys from March 2005 to March 2006. The countries covered by the surveys were: Botswana, Ghana, Lesotho, Malawi, Mali, Namibia, Nigeria, South Africa, Uganda, Zambia and Zimbabwe. The surveys have since included Benin, Cape Verde, Kenya, Madagascar, Mozambique and Senegal. The minimum sample size in each country is 1 200, which its experts explain is sufficient to produce a confidence interval of plus or minus 3% points at a confidence level of 95% (Bratton & Cho: 2006).

It may perplex observers that despite the gravity of HIV/AIDS, poor people, who would normally be considered the most affected by the epidemic, regard the epidemic as less important in relation to other concerns such as food security or access to medical care for other debilitating illnesses (TB, malaria, cholera). Understandably, citizens in a country like Senegal or other low-prevalence West African countries such as Ghana are unlikely to place AIDS as their main priority in the face of immediate threats to their wellbeing (unemployment, crime, food insecurity, etc). Their counterparts in the SADC region will similarly respond to questions on less stigmatising diseases more openly. Cholera, malaria and TB decimate their victims much faster than the slow onslaught characterised by the array of opportunistic infections that define AIDS. A cholera epidemic for example will constitute a clear and present danger to society requiring swift policy responses from the government given also the international embarrassment that comes with this so-called "disease of poverty".

> **Poor people regard the epidemic as less important in relation to other concerns such as food security.**

Indeed, it is also conceivable that not many people would wish to associate themselves with an epidemic that attracts discrimination even through mere perception of illness. It is quite possible that the majority of the respondents did not wish to be seen to be ill, as a demonstration of concern about AIDS might imply. We have seen from Idasa's multi-country studies that political elites will not disclose their HIV status unless it is sero-negative. This "secrecy" is what renders public opinion surveys in matters of a deeply personal nature limited in their effectiveness.

The flip side of this discussion is that in the same survey, two-thirds of all adult respondents in 2005 on average thought their governments had performed well on AIDS. Afrobarometer reports that respondents in 2005 gave governments better

Figure 4.6: Voter turnout as a percentage of registerd voters (2004-2006)

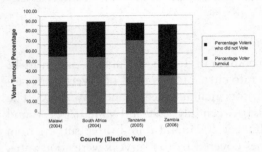

Figure 4.7: Voter turnout as a percentage of voting age population (2004-2006)

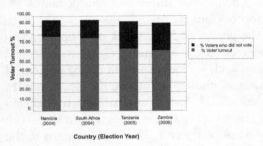

grades (70%) for HIV/AIDS management than for any other social policy.[81]

The flow of optimism obviously does not reflect reality as rightly indicated by the Afrobarometer. As already discussed, the incidence of AIDS continues to rise even as its prevalence in some countries, such as Uganda, Kenya and Zimbabwe, is reportedly declining. The Afrobarometer attributes this to possible misinformation due to the relatively low infection rates in West Africa; the availability of ART; and persistence of social taboos amongst the local communities and political elites alike.

We should not perhaps underestimate the impact of the introduction of ART on local communities as this represents a major departure from the 1980s/90s scenario when AIDS was seen to represent a swift progression to a painful death, encouraging increasing abandonment of sufferers. And while politicians are notable absentees in the VCT circles, they still dominate the airwaves with pronouncements on government delivery of drugs and PLWHAs-friendly policies at both national and regional levels.

The accompanying evidence of ART on the ground, albeit limited, could be having profound effects on perceptions regarding governments' commitment (although donor funding also plays a significant part in this). As stated earlier, even as the incidence of HIV is rising, the number of people on ART in low- and middle-income countries almost doubled from 720 000 to 1.3 million in 2005, the year in which Afrobarometer concluded its round three.

CHAPTER FIVE: OBSERVATIONS AND RECOMMENDATIONS

There are a number of worrying revelations in this study: the large number of younger voters who have died in a space of five years in South Africa; the rise in deaths amongst MPs in Malawi, Tanzania, Zambia and Zimbabwe and more generally; the loss of representation attributed to these deaths; the effect on the capacity of parliament and potential effect on institutional memory; the impact on small or under-resourced opposition parties and the implications for democratic accountability. There should also be concerns about the deep-seated stigma and discrimination amongst the political elite in several countries under study and finally the economic costs generated by HIV/AIDS through multiple by-elections all of which provide a strong basis to argue for new interventions to redress the situation. Such interventions will need to transcend traditional health approaches and in fact challenge us to deal with our democratic deficits in tandem with AIDS activities. In that sense, the following proposals and observations may serve to help countries absorb the shocks of HIV/AIDS as well as consolidate their electoral profiles:

1. ELECTORAL ENGINEERING AND PUBLIC CHOICE

Firstly, there is a need to modify the FPTP system given its susceptibility to HIV/AIDS. This could mean either waiving the requirement for by-elections or adopting a PR system. This route is of course not as straightforward as it sounds. Adopting a PR system comes with concerns around poor accountability as MPs will not be directly elected by the people. The MMP system provides some modicum of compromise but is itself quite vulnerable to by-elections as demonstrated in Lesotho. Electoral reform is a long-term enterprise requiring wide consultation through a constitutional review process and depending on how soon political actors can reach consensus on AIDS as one of the key threats to a sustainable democracy, it may be a while before we actually see any changes. Our recommendation, given the complexities and multiple considerations for reform that need equitable attention, is that countries operating the FPTP, MMP and Parallel systems may need to modify their systems to include MP substitution. A viable option would be to simply allow political parties to replace the deceased through appointment.

We noted that electoral systems also have impacts on human development. Majoritarian systems record comparatively lower human development levels than the proportional models. This further challenges nation-states to carefully consider their choices. In the age of AIDS it is prudent to tailor new electoral models toward a goal that seeks to contribute to the upliftment of people's general welfare. In this regard, experts have to assess all imperatives in order to arrive at a home-grown model.

2. POLITICAL PARTIES

Secondly, it is certain that there is no place for people living with HIV in political party leadership. The stigma and discrimination that is now known to exist amongst the political elite will require innovative solutions. Failure to address this situation may compromise the many efforts by AIDS service organisations aimed at building a strong leadership required to tackle the problem of AIDS. New strategies need to be adopted that encourage political parties to deliberately infuse PLWHAs into their ranks. This is particularly possible in countries using the PR and MMP systems. However, FPTP countries could also exploit the slots for nominated MPs to appoint PLWHAs. The presence of dominant parties such as the ANC in South Africa and the Botswana Democratic Party (BDP) in Botswana, which are not in immediate threat of losing an election, provides a genuine opportunity to dramatically impact on stigma and discrimination in politics and society in general by adopting a person living with HIV/AIDS as a candidate for parliament or local government.

> Training and knowledge-building is needed for parliamentarians to enable them to act on political, social and economic challenges.

At a more strategic level, political parties will need to develop succession plans where none exist and initiate workplace programmes with strong information, education and communication components on the political, economic and social dynamics of AIDS in addition to the personal health matters. There is now evidence in South Africa for instance of the IFP embarking on an elaborate HIV/AIDS programme aimed at providing care and support to affected members, details of which were not available at the time of writing.

3. PARLIAMENTS

It is surprising that despite what might be described as a very noticeable trend of deaths from undisclosed illnesses amongst MPs, none of the parliaments have discussed the effects of HIV/AIDS on parliamentary capacity and institutional memory. Instead debates have focused on society at large. Parliamentary bodies are best placed to commission internal investigative processes on MP attrition and solicit appropriate strategic support from experts in civil society organisations (CSOs), academia and the development sector. Workplace policies with strong all-encompassing information, education and communication strategies need to be instituted to help develop pools of AIDS competent MPs.

Training and knowledge-building is needed for parliamentarians to enable them to act on the political, social and economic challenges faced by their constituencies and employ that knowledge in their oversight functions. We take cognisance of the fact that not every parliamentarian will treat HIV/AIDS as a priority. There is therefore a need to identify champions in parliamentary bodies who would form the core of strategic parliamentary interventions.

4. PUBLIC PARTICIPATION IN PARLIAMENTARY PROCESS

Parliaments at present are generally quite removed from the people. They are Europeanised institutions whose language of instruction is often restricted to people with a western education. Parliaments are in addition located in national capitals and will be completely out of reach of ordinary rural and peri-urban folk. Even where they are accessible, entering the public gallery of parliament as a passive observer requires certain adherence to dress codes, not to mention there is limited space available. We would encourage greater interaction between parliamentarians and PLWHAs and other CSOs to help define and solve the problem. Issues such as discrimination in politics, employment and financial services require legislative interventions and are fundamental to reversing the impact of HIV/AIDS. At present, few parliaments have the budget to hold public hearings and these will normally be held by specific committees.[82] But public hearings remain important in engaging the broader public on matters of HIV/AIDS and governance and therefore funds should be set aside to facilitate them.

5. LEGISLATIVE PROTECTION OF PLWHAS

While parliaments have contributed to a legislative response by instituting provisions for the criminalisation of wilful transmission of HIV, there is clearly a need for further state interventions in ensuring that discriminatory practices in the employment, banking industries and for that matter in the political sphere are eliminated. Exclusionary tendencies are deeply entrenched in the practices of insurance companies, employment agencies and lending organisations and these replicate themselves in the area of electoral politics.

Underlining the fact that HIV/AIDS is a manageable ailment, and therefore requires accommodative considerations by all sectors through a well-structured legislative intervention, could help minimise institutional stigma and discrimination across many fields including politics.

6. VOTER PARTICIPATION

The research suggests further that there are roles for the EMBs in the HIV/AIDS field. The impact of stigma and discrimination on participation, though only indicative in rural South Africa, deserves attention as it may be more extensive than this study suggests, with ramifications for the involvement of individuals infected and affected in politics. EMBs could assist by incorporating non-discriminatory messages in their voter education campaigns which encourage more people to participate in elections and ensure there is tolerance to a greater degree of people who are ill. Only the Zanzibar Electoral Commission encouraged political parties to deploy AIDS awareness messages during the 2005 election in Tanzania.[84] Setting up special voting mechanisms for the disadvantaged might also be a consideration as is the case in South Africa. Such facilities should not be exclusively tailored to PLWHAs to avoid accentuating stigma and discrimination; they should rather seek to engage all persons with disability and those challenged by ill health, among others.

7. ELECTORAL GOVERNANCE

Countries in Africa that do not have institutionalised and directly compatible citizen and voter registration systems will be unable to determine the extent to which HIV/AIDS has undermined their political institutions. This will impact on their electoral planning and more generally on their long-term developmental visions. We can see from the case of Malawi that doubts about the size of the voters' roll can contribute to weak political mandates and instability. Investment in new technologies is recommended to ensure timeous deletion of dead voters to avert unnecessary post-election conflict.

8. AIDS SERVICE ORGANISATIONS

It is time that traditional NGOs dealing with HIV/AIDS took on board new research perspectives that could inform their actions toward the MDG targets. One of the lessons from this study is that AIDS is not a problem of one specific industry, requiring only sector-specific responses. It challenges us to continually review our strategies based on fresh knowledge. Donor support for innovative social and political research may prove important in galvanising the key policy actors who, from time to time, appear to lose sight of the relevance of HIV/AIDS as a long-term adversary.

Appendix: Impact of HIV/AIDS on democratic governance (adapted, POKU: 2007)

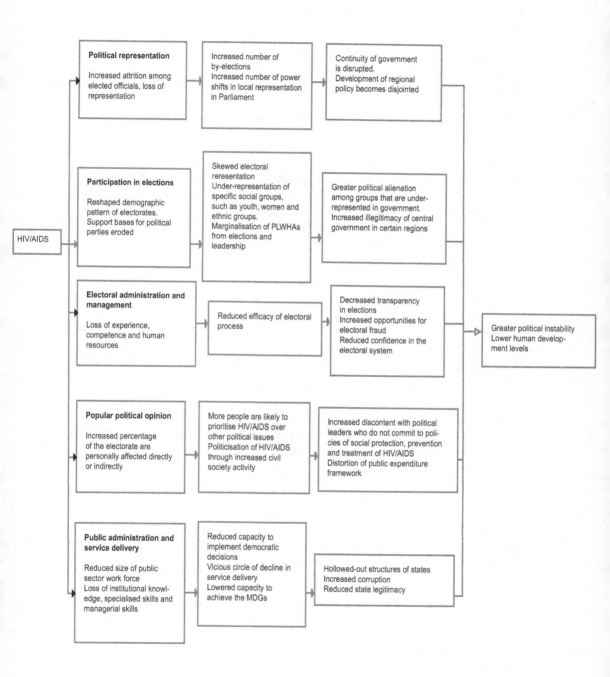

ENDNOTES

1 Meehan (1998; p 136, Para 1) asserts that: "what identifies a reasoned choice or action is the element of deliberate weighing or comparing of outcomes, balancing the benefits to humans of selecting each of the alternatives".

2 See Chirambo K & Caesar M (Eds) (2003); AIDS and Governance in Southern Africa: Emerging Theories and Perspective. Cape Town: Idasa.

3 Also known as Low Income Countries Under Stress (LUCUS) that are defined by weak policies, institutions and governance.

4 Youde J. (2001) All the Voters will be Dead: HIV/AIDS and Democratic Legitimacy and Stability in Africa (Iowa).

5 Lately, social researchers in Africa seem to agree that without the extended family and kinship systems, the impact of HIV/AIDS on African societies would have been much worse. Africa hosts 95% of the 13 million so-called AIDS orphans. See Matshalaga N. & Powell G., (2002) Mass Orphanhood in the Era of HIV/AIDS: Bold Support for Alleviation of Poverty and Education may Avoid a Social Disaster. http://www.pubmedcentral.nih.gov/articlerender.fcgi?artid=1122118 & IRIN news report: Malawi: Illegal Orphanages Mushroom: http://www.irinnews.org/report.aspx?reportid=61374

6 www.cosatu.org.za/congress/conggg/all-res.htm

7 Author's italicisation.

8 Parsons W. (1995) argues that public policy has to do with those spheres which could be designated as "public"; that are held as common to all; the dimension of human activity which is regarded as requiring governmental or social regulation or intervention or at least common action.

9 Author's italicisation.

10 Statement by Peter Piot, Director, UNAIDS, UN University, 2 October, 2001. http://www.africaaction.org/docs01/piot0110.htm

11 For instance the SADC Declaration on Gender and Development of 1997 seeks gender balance, recognising the disadvantaged position in decision-making mechanisms, concerns arising from the Beijing Declaration and Platform for Action. See The SADC MPs Companion on Gender and Development in Southern Africa (2002) SARDC/SADC-PF.

12 Author's italisation.

13 In *Deepening Democracy in a Fragmented World. UNDP Human Development Report 2002.* New York, available at www.undp.org p: 51, the UNDP states that "from a human development perspective, good governance is democratic governance".

14 See Matlosa K., Chiroro B., Letsholo S., (2007): Politics of Electoral System Reform and Democratisation: Contemporary Trends in Southern Africa. EISA; Johannesburg. Conference paper.

15 Reynolds et al (2005): Electoral System Design: the International IDEA Handbook: IDEA: Stockholm.

16 The SADC MPs Companion on Gender and Development in Southern Africa. Harare (2002): SARDC/SADC Parliamentary Forum.

17 Zambia National Women's Lobby Group: End of Year Report January-December 2001; Submitted to Netherlands Embassy; p 19.

18 http://www.statistics.gov.uk/census2001/cb_8.asp. The resolution of Cosatu's 8th National Congress in 2003 sought to introduce a 65% constituency-based system combined with 33% proportional representation.

19 SADC Parliamentary Forum: (2001) Norms and Standards for Elections in the SADC Region: Windhoek: SADC-PF.

20 SADC and International Cooperating Partners: Framework on Regional Support to HIV and AIDS in Southern Africa. 2006.

21 Tredoux C. & Durrheim explain that "Variables are measured entities (or attributes of entities that

can take on different values i.e. as height, weight. Independent variables are variables that are pre-sumed to affect or determine other variables. Dependent variables are affected or determined by inde-pendent variables" pp 9-14).

22   Barnett and Whiteside explain that the epidemic comes in successive waves, the first being HIV infec-tion; followed several years later by a wave of opportunistic infections and finally a third wave of ill-ness and death.

23   UNAIDS/WHO global reports (2002-2005); Iliffe J. (2006) The African AIDS Epidemic. A History. Oxford. James Curray Ltd.

24   Daniel Halperin & Helen Epstein (2006): The Role of Multiple Concurrent Partnerships and Lack of Male Circumcision.

25   SADC and International Cooperating Partners: Framework on Regional Support to HIV and AIDS in Southern Africa. 2006.

26   Life expectancy at birth is the average number of years a person can expect to live at current levels of mortality. These estimates are the outcome of modelling by the UN and national estimates for some countries may differ significantly, e.g. Botswana estimates its life expectancy to be 55 years compared to the UN figure of 36.

27   Workshop report on Human Mobility, Migration and HIV/AIDS, Idasa 2002. www.idasa.org

28   The factors are prevalent in all of the countries in the region to varying degrees.

29   Daniel Halperin & Helen Epstein (2006): The Role of Multiple Concurrent Partnerships and Lack of Male Circumcision. www.healthdev.org/eforums/editor/assets/accelerating-prevention/daniel_halper-in's% 20key_paper_FINAL%20 VERSION.pdf

30   According to expert sources, both types have a range of sub-types. They will both be transmitted sexually, through blood and through mother to child transmission and will cause "clinically indistin-guishable AIDS". Experts note however that HIV-2 is less easily transmitted and the period between initial infection and illness is longer in the case of HIV-2. HIV-2 is concentrated in West Africa and rarely found elsewhere. The pre-dominant virus is HIV-1(www. avert.org).

31   In a number of countries in the region, adult women are still considered to be "minors" for purposes of inheritance and owning property. This makes them highly dependent on male relatives (husbands, fathers and brothers).

32   Chirambo K. & Caesar M (Eds) (2003): AIDS and Governance in Southern Africa; Emerging Theories and Perspectives. Idasa: Cape Town.

33   Daniel Halperin & Helen Epstein (2006): Tthe Role of Multiple Concurrent Partnerships and Lack of Male Circumcision. www.healthdev.org/eforums/editor/assets/accelerating-prevention/daniel_halper-in's% 20key_paper_FINAL%20 VERSION.pdf

34   Crush J., Frayne B., & Grant M. (2006) Linking Migration, HIV/AIDS and Urban Food Security in Southern and Eastern Africa. RENEWAL. IFPRI, SAMP. www.queensu.ca/samp. Crush et al caution against stigmatising migrants as bearers of disease and enacting restrictive laws in that regard: rather, there is need to direct HIV/AIDS interventions such as education, prevention, voluntary counselling and testing, and treatment and care as part of a holistic strategy of dealing with the pandemic.

35   IRIN: Southern Africa: Conflict, Development and Natural Disasters Fuel Internal Displacement. 14 February 2006, United Nations Office for the Coordination of Humanitarian Affairs-inte-grated Regional Information Networks (IRIN).http://www.reliefweb.int/rw/rwb.nsf/db900sid/KHII-6M25GM?Opendocument

36   Niedan C., (2006): West African Conflict Roots Examined. 10/3/03. http://www.pittnews.com/home/index.cfm?event

37   IRIN reports that: "experts have long assumed that the violence, wide-scale rape and refugee crises are the inevitable by-product of war that fuel HIV/AIDS epidemics, but an analysis of HIV prevalence surveys from seven Sub-Saharan African countries with similar recent histories found no evidence that higher HIV infection rates accompany conflict. The study is available at (http://www.thelancet.

com/journals/lancet/article/PIIS0140673607610150/fullt

38 IRIN report at ⟨http://www.thelancet.com/journals/lancet/article/PIIS0140673607610150/fullt

39 Halperin and Helen Epstein differentiate the two practices as such: the tendency to have one relative-ly long term (a few months or longer) partner after another (concurrent partnership)…or more "once off" casual and commercial sexual encounters that occur everywhere" (serial monogamy).

40 Niang I (2008) Re-Thinking AIDS and Governance; the case of Senegal. In Chirambo K (ed). 2008. *The Political Cost of AIDS in Africa: Evidence from Six Countries. Cape Town:* Idasa.

41 International HIV/AIDS Alliance.http://aidsalliance.org/sw44583.asp?usepf=true

42 International HIV/AIDS Alliance.http://aidsalliance.org/sw44583.asp?usepf=true

43 See also, Information and Library Services Exchange. http://www.kit.nl/exchange/html/2001_2_har-nessing_senegal_s_ap.asp

44 Southern African News Features no. 39, August 2007: SARDC.

45 Chirambo K & McCullum H. Reporting Elections in Southern Africa: A Media Handbook: SARDC 2000.

46 Ibid.

47 SADC regional Human Development Report 2000; UNDP; SADC;SAPES Trust

48 Human Development Indicators in the SADC Region, DPRU Policy Brief No. 01/p13, May 2001

49 Southern African News Features no. 39, August 2007: SARDC

50 SADC Update, 04/18/01. http://www.africa.upenn.edu/Urgent_Action/apic-041801.html

51 The focus areas of harmonisation were:
- Care and treatment including the use of ARVs
- Nutrition, nutritional therapies and traditional herbs
- Human resource needs in all sectors in the context of HIV/AIDS
- Regional HIV/AIDS issues such as migrant population/mobile labour, refugees and displaced populations
- Harmonisation of procedures, regulations and laws of transit at borders and ports
- Bulk procurement of drugs and medical supplies of HIV/AIDS
- Regional guidelines for clinical trials
- Guidelines for programme intervention in High Transmission Areas such as border sites and high traf-fic sites
- Sustenance of human capital in the context of HIV/AIDS in the region
- Policy guidelines on how to increase access to care and treatment of the most vulnerable social groups
- Mainstreaming

52 Forthcoming: Impact of AIDS on National Budgets in Africa: Cape Town: Idasa.

53 Scaling Up HIV Prevention, Treatment Care and Support (2006). UN.

54 Chipika J. T.(2007) Current Macroeconomic Frameworks, Challenges and Alternatives for the Attainment of the Millennium Development Goals: http://www.sarpn.org.za/document/d0002654/index.php

55 Cheema, G.S. (2000) in Good Governance: A Path to Poverty Eradication; defines governance as " a set of values, policies and institutions by which a society manages its economic, political and social processes at all levels through interaction among government, civil society and private sector," UNDP.

56 Author's italicisation.

57 Moeletsi Mbeki's address to the opening of the European Association of Centres of African Studies Conference, Leiden University in the Netherlands, 11 to 14 July 2007. Mbeki is deputy chair of the South African Institute of International Affairs. He refers also to the post-colonial era as a period of partnership between western donors and emergent African dictators in plundering mineral and intel-lectual wealth and the destruction of indigenous institutions that were critical to political and social mobilisation; the African nationalist party was one significant casualty.

58 ZHDR (2002) Human Development Report, Oxford: Oxford University Press. First quoted Strand P., Matlosa K., Strode A., & Chirambo K (2005) HIV/AIDS and Democratic Governance in South

Africa: Illustrating the Impact on the Electoral Process. Idasa: Cape Town. With thanks to Richard Calland, manager of Idasa's Economic Governance Programme (EGP) and staff for additional input into the nine principles.

59   Statement by Peter Piot, Executive Director of UNAIDS 2001. http://www.africaaction.org/docs01/piot0110.htm

60   See Niang et al (Forthcoming); HIV/AIDS and Democratic Governance in Senegal: Illustrating the Impact on Electoral Processes. Cape Town. Idasa: "These rates, considered as relatively low in the Sub-Saharan African context, however conceal substantial disparities between the various regions of the country".

61   Barnett and Whiteside explain that the epidemic comes in successive waves, the first being HIV infection; followed several years later by a wave of opportunistic infections and finally a third wave of illness and death.

62   Mattes R. & Strand P (2007) AIDS Impact Research at DARU: HIV/AIDS and Society: Building a Community of Practice. Cape Town.

63   In 2005, the speaker of the National Assembly of Malawi was flown to South Africa for further medical treatment. Similarly, leading politicians from Zambia often access medical aid from South Africa or in Europe.

64   Sachs M. (2002) By Elections in 2001: A Statistical Review. UMRABULO. Issue number 14 in April ANC. www.anc.org.za/ancdocs/pubs/umrabulo/umrabulo14/elections.html

65   By-elections costs include, transport, printing of ballot papers, allowances or election officers, presiding officers, tents, lighting, distribution of voters' registers, transport (air and land), among others.

66   http://concourt.law.wits.ac.za/judges/jdcameron.html

67   http://www.beatit.co.za/episode9.php.

68   According to the Electoral Commission of Zambia's Deputy Director, Priscilla Isaacs, (telephone interview, 2004): and official statement to Idasa released in 2007.

69   Using the rate of 1 USD= 6.9637 rand, September 25th, 2007

70   By-elections costs include, transport, printing of ballot papers, allowances or election officers, presiding officers, tents, lighting, distribution of voters' registers, transport (air and land), among others.

71   Tsie B., (2000). Electoral Sustainability and the Cost of Development. Johannesburg: EISA

72   Using the rate of 1 USD= 6.9637 rand, September 25th, 2007

73   Chirambo K (2006): Democratisation in the Age of HIV/AIDS: Understanding the Political Implications. Cape Town: Idasa.

74   Academy International Affairs Working Paper Series: (2006) Mitigating HIV/AIDS Impacts on Teachers and Administrators in Sub-Saharan Africa. Washington: www.napawash.org

75   The actual size of the voters' roll is not known due to discrepancies in both citizen and voter registration. Malawi does not have an established citizen registration and identification system and has therefore found it difficult to determine just how many of its people are of voting age. Malawi's voters' roll is hence not regularly updated. In 1999, a total of 5 071 822 voters were registered (national population of 11 million) and of these 2 417 713 were registered in the southern region, 1 975 203 in the central region and 678 906 in the northern region. However in April 2004, the MEC announced that 6 668 839 voters had registered for the May 18, 2004 presidential and parliamentary elections.54 These figures were challenged by opposition political parties and other institutions with the National Statistical Office taking the lead. It described the figure as "bogus" because it did not conform to the country's natural demographic trends. The result of Malawi's problematic voters' roll is a weak mandate for the new government and post-election conflict over outcomes. Malawi has been preoccupied with impeachment tensions since the last presidential polls.

76   Some records show a figure of 6.7 million registered at this time.

77   Ibid

78   Kapembwa Simbao, (former) Deputy Minister of Health, Zambia, in his opening speech at the Idasa/FODEP/INESOR policy forum on AIDS and elections, 2005.

79 Interview on 13 April 2006.
80 Interview on 20 April 2006.
81 Bratton M., & Cho W., (2006) Working Paper No.60. Where is Africa Going? Views from Below. A Compendium of Trends in Public Opinion in 12 Countries, 1999-2006. Cape Town: Idasa/ CDD/MSU
82 Caesar M., & Myburg M (2006) Parliaments, Politics and AIDS; Comparative Study of Five African Countries. Cape Town: Idasa.
83 Zanzibar and Tanganyika form one state under the Union of the Republic of Tanzania.

REFERENCES

BOOKS

Bang P. H. (2003) Governance as Social and Political Communication. Manchester University Press.

Barnett T. and Whiteside A. (2002) HIV/AIDS in the Twenty-First Century: Disease and Globalisation. New York: Palgrave Macmillan.

Braman S. (2003) Communication Researchers and Policy-making. Massachusetts Institute of Technology.

Bratton M. & Cho W. (2006) Working Paper No.60. Where is Africa Going? Views from Below. A Compendium of Trends in Public Opinion in 12 Countries, 1999-2006. Cape Town: Idasa/ CDD/MSU

Bumler J. G. (1996) Introduction to Political Communication. Module Two: Unit 12. MA in Mass Communications. Centre for Mass Communication Research. Leicester University.

Caesar M., & Myburg M (2006) Parliaments, Politics and AIDS; Comparative Study of Five African Countries. Cape Town: Idasa.

Cheema, G. S. (2000) In Good Governance: A Path to Poverty Eradication. New York: United Nations Development Programme (UNDP).

Chirambo K. & McCullum H. (2000) Reporting Elections in Southern Africa: A Media Handbook: SARDC.

Chirambo K. (2003) Impact of HIV/AIDS on Electoral Processes in Southern Africa. Presentation to the UNDP/Idasa Satellite Conference, Nairobi, September. Idasa.

Chirambo K. and Caesar M. (eds) (2003) HIV/AIDS and Governance in Southern Africa: Emerging Theories and Perspectives. Cape Town: Idasa.

Chirambo, K. (2004) AIDS and Electoral Democracy: Implications for Participation, Political Stability and Accountability in Southern Africa. Johannesburg: EISA.

Chirambo K. (2005) AIDS & Electoral Democracy: Insights into Impacts on Africa's Democratic Institutions. Pretoria: Institute for Democracy in South Africa. Cape Town: Idasa.

Chirambo K. (2006) Democratisation in the Age of HIV/AIDS: Understanding the Political Implications. Cape Town: Idasa.

Chirambo K., Nel N. and Erasmus C. (2003) Zambia Presidential, Parliamentary and Local Government Elections, 2001; Evaluation of Impact of Donor Investment. Pretoria: Idasa.

De Renzio P. (2004) The Challenge of Absorptive Capacity: Will Lack of Absorptive Capacity Prevent Effective Uuse of Additional Aid Resources in Pursuit of the MDGs? Report on seminar at DFID, Overseas Development Institute, London.

Fay B. (1993) Elements of Critical Social Science. In Hammersley, Social Research: Philosophy, Politics and Practice. London: SAGE.

Gassner M., Onhiveros U. and Verardi V. (2005) Electoral Systems and Human Development. Journal of Human Development Alternative Economics in Action. Vol 7 No 1, March 2006.

Halloran J. (1995) Media Research as Social Science. Module One: Unit 2, in MA in Mass Communications, Centre for Mass Communications Research: Leicester University.

Hammerssley M. (1993) Social Research: Philosophy, Politics and Practice. London: SAGE.

Hansen A., Cottle S., Negrine R. & Newbold C. (1998) Mass Communication Research Methods. London: Macmillan Press Ltd.

Hunter S. (2003) Who Cares? AIDS in Africa. New York. Palgrave Macmillan.

Hyden G., Court J. & Mease K. (2004) Making Sense of Governance: Empirical Evidence from 16 Countries. London: Rienner.

Illiffe J. (2006) The African AIDS Pandemic: A History. Oxford: James A Curray Ltd. University.

Lodge T. (2004) Handbook of South African Electoral Laws and Regulations. Johannesburg: EISA.

Matlosa K., Chiroro B. & Letsholo S. (2007) Politics of Electoral System Reform and Democratisation: Contemporary Trends in Southern Africa. Johannesburg EISA, conference paper.

Meehan E. J. (1988) The Thinking Game: A Guide to Effective Study. New Jersey; Chatam House.

Ndhlovu N. & Daswa R.(2006) Review of progress on the Comprehensive Plan for HIV and AIDS for South Africa. Occasional papers. AIDS Budget Unit, Idasa, Cape Town.

Parsons W. (1995) Public Policy: An Introduction to the Theory and Practice of Policy Analysis. Cheltenham: Edward Edgar Publishing Ltd.

Poku N. (2007) PowerPoint presentation to Idasa's second Governance and AIDS Forum, Cape Town: May 22-24.

Reynolds A., Reilly B. & Ellis A. (eds) (2005) Electoral System Design: The International IDEA Handbook. Stockholm: IDEA.

Simbao K. (2005) Opening speech at the Idasa/FODEP/INESOR policy forum on AIDS and Elections, quoted in Chirambo K. AIDS & Electoral Democracy: Insights into Impacts on Africa's Democratic Institutions. Cape Town: Idasa.

Strand P., Matlosa K., Strode A. & Chirambo K. (2005) HIV/AIDS and Democratic Governance in South Africa: Illustrating the Impact on Electoral Processes. Cape Town: Idasa.

Tredoux C. & Durrheim (eds) (2002) Numbers, Hypotheses & Conclusions: A Course in Statistics for the Social Sciences. Cape Town: UCT Press.

Tsie B. (2000). Electoral Sustainability and the Cost of Development. Johannesburg: EISA.

Youde J. (2001) All the Voters Will be Dead: HIV/AIDS and Democratic Legitimacy and Stability in Africa. Iowa.

OFFICIAL SOURCES

CHGA (2004), Q & A on HIV/AIDS and Governance in Africa. Addis Ababa: Commission for HIV/AIDS Governance in Africa/Economic Commission for Africa.

DPRU. (2001) Human Development Indicators in the SADC Region.

EISA (2003) Principles for Election Management, Monitoring and Observation in the SADC Region. Johannesburg: Electoral Commissions Forum/Electoral Institute of Southern Africa.

IDEA. (2000) The Functioning and Funding of Political Parties in the SADC Region: An Overview; Conference on Sustainable Democratic Institutions in Southern Africa. Stockholm: IDEA.

Human Development Indicators in the SADC Region, DPRU Policy Brief No. 01/p13, May 2001

Idasa/HEARD/DARU. (2002) AIDS and Democracy Workshop for Researchers Report.

NAC. (2004) The HIV/AIDS Epidemic in Zambia: Where are we now? Where are we going? Lusaka: September.

NAC. (2004) HIV/AIDS Communication Strategy. Lusaka: May.

National Intelligence Council. (2005) Mapping Sub-Saharan Africa's Future, Conference Report.

Nelson Mandela/HSRC Study of HIV/AIDS, (2002) Cape Town: Human Sciences Research Council.

Nepad. (2003) Nepad Health Strategy. Pretoria: Nepad.

NIMD. (2004) Institutional Development Handbook. A Framework for Democratic Party-Building. Hague: Netherlands Institute for Multiparty Democracy.

Principles for Election Management, Monitoring and Observation in the SADC Region. (2003) Johannesburg: EISA.

SADC Human Development Report. (2000) Challenges, Opportunities for Regional Integration. UNDP/SAPES.

SADC (2003) HIV/AIDS Strategic Framework and Programme of Action 2003-2007: Managing the HIV/AIDS Pandemic in Southern African Development Community, July, 2003

SADC and International Cooperating Partners: Framework on Regional Support to HIV and AIDS in Southern Africa. (2006).

SADC Parliamentary Forum. (2001) Norms and Standards for Elections in the SADC Region. Windhoek: SADC-PF.

SARDC. (1999) Zambia Democracy Fact file. Harare: SARDC.

SARDC/SADC-Parliamentary Forum. (2002) The SADC MPs Companion on Gender and Development in southern Africa. Harare: SARDC.

SARDC. (2007) Southern African News Features no. 39, August.

Scaling Up HIV Prevention, Treatment Care and Support. (2006). UN.

UNAIDS/WHO global reports (2002-2005).

UNDP. (2002) Deepening Democracy in a Fragmented World. Human Development Report 2002. New York: United Nations Development Programme. available at www.undp.org

UNDP. (2000) Zimbabwe Human Development Report. Governance. UNDP.

Zambia National Women's Lobby Group. (2001) End of Year Report January – December; Submitted to Netherlands Embassy; p 19.

UNECA. (2005) Striving for Good Governance in Africa. Addis Ababa: United Nations Economic Commission for Africa.

WHO/UNAIDS. (2006) Global Report 2002-2005.

NEWSPAPER ARTICLES

New York Times (2001) AIDS Permeates Uganda Politics Too. March 12, Ian Fisher.

Star (2005) 11 Teachers a Day Die of AIDS, April 1; Ndivhuwo Khangale & Sapa

INTERVIEW

Priscilla Isaacs, (telephone interview, 2004)

ARTICLES FROM WEBSITES

Academy International Affairs Working Paper Series. (2006) Mitigating HIV/AIDS Impacts on Teachers and Administrators in Sub-Saharan Africa. Washington: www.napawash.org

Chipika J. T (2007) Current Macroeconomic Frameworks, Challenges and Alternatives for the Attainment of the Millennium Development Goals. http://www.sarpn.org.za/document/d0002654/index.php International HIV/AIDS Alliance.http://aidsalliance.org/sw44583.asp?usepf=true

Crush J., Frayne B. & Grant M. (2006) Linking Migration, HIV/AIDS and Urban Food Security in Southern and Eastern Africa. RENEWAL. IFPRI, SAMP. http://www.queensu.ca/samp

Halperin D. & Epstein H. (2006) The Role of Multiple Concurrent Partnerships and Lack of Male Circumcision. www.healthdev.org/eforums/editor/assets/accelerating-prevention/daniel_halperin's%20key_paper_FINAL%20 VERSION.pdf

Information and Library Services Exchange. http://www.kit.nl/exchange/html/2001_2_harnessing_senegal_s_ap.asp

IRIN news report: Malawi: Illegal Orphanages Mushroom. http://www.irinnews.org/report.aspx?reportid=61374

Matshalaga N. & Powell G. (2002) Mass Orphanhood in the Era of HIV/AIDS: Bold Support for Alleviation of Poverty and Education May Avert a Social Disaster. http://www.pubmedcentral.nih.gov/articlerender.fcgi?artid=1122118

Mayntz, R. (2003), From government to governance: Political steering in modern societies. Presented at the Summer Academy on IPP at Wuerzburg, September 7-11 2003. http://www.ioew.de/gov.../SuA2Mayntz.pdf.
http://www.ioew.de/governance/english/veranstaltungen/Summer_Academies/SuA2Mayntz.pdf

Niedan C. (2006) West African Conflict Roots Examined. (2003).
http://www.pittnews.com/home/index.cfm?event

Panos/UNICEF. (2004). Stigma, HIV/AIDS and Prevention of Mother-to Child Transmission: A Pilot Study in Zambia, Ukraine, India and Burkina Faso.

Sachs M. (2002) By-Elections in 2001: A Statistical Review. UMRABULO. Issue number 14 in April ANC.
www.anc.org.za/ancdocs/pubs/umrabulo/umrabulo14/elections.html

SADC Update, 04/18/01. http://www.africa.upenn.edu/Urgent_Action/apic-041801.html

Statement by Peter Piot, Executive Director of UNAIDS 2001.
http://www.africaaction.org/docs01/piot0110.htm

UNAIDS; Report on the Global AIDS epidemic (2006) UNAIDS.
http://www.unaids.org/en/hiv_data/2006globalreport/default.asp

Willan S. (2004) Recent Changes in the South African Government's HIV/AIDS Policy and its Implementation. HEARD; University of Natal.
http://http://afraf.oxfordjournals.org/cgi/content/abstract/103/410/109?etoc